MW00676978

BABY
SKIN

ALSO BY NELSON LEE NOVICK, M.D.

Saving Face
Skin Care for Teens
Super Skin

BABY SKIN

A LEADING DERMATOLOGIST'S GUIDE TO INFANT AND CHILDHOOD SKIN CARE

NELSON LEE NOVICK, M.D.

CLARKSON POTTER/PUBLISHERS
NEW YORK

Publisher's Note: This book contains recommendations to be followed within the context of an overall health-care program. However, not all recommendations are designed for all individuals. While the book discusses certain issues and choices regarding skin care, it is not intended as a substitute for professional medical advice. Before following these or any other health-care recommendations, a physician should be consulted.

Many products mentioned in this book are trademarks of their respective companies. Every effort has been made to identify these trademarks by initial capitalization. Should there be any errors or omissions in this respect, we shall be pleased to make the necessary corrections in future editions.

Copyright © 1991 by Nelson Lee Novick
All rights reserved. No part of this book may be reproduced or transmitted in any form or by any means, electronic or mechanical, including photocopying, recording, or by any information storage and retrieval system, without permission in writing from the publisher.

Published by Clarkson N. Potter, Inc., 201 East 50th Street, New York, New York 10022. Member of the Crown Publishing Group.

CLARKSON POTTER, POTTER, and colophon are trademarks of Clarkson N. Potter, Inc.

Manufactured in the United States of America

LIBRARY OF CONGRESS CATALOGING-IN-PUBLICATION DATA
Novick, Nelson Lee.
Baby skin : a leading dermatologist's guide to infant and childhood skin care / by Nelson Lee Novick.—1st ed.
p. cm.
Includes index.
1. Skin—Care and hygiene. 2. Infants—Care. 3. Child care.
I. Title.
RL87.N67 1991
649'.4—dc20
ISBN 0-517-58422-0

10   9   8   7   6   5   4   3   2   1

First Edition

To my wife and dearest friend, Meryl,
who enabled me to complete this work by
quietly shouldering so many additional burdens
and responsibilities. And to my five sons,
Yoni, Yoel, Ariel, Donny, and Avi, who add a
dimension to my life that makes it all worthwhile.

———

Special thanks to my office manager,
Barbara Jerabek, for the idea for the book
and for the countless hours she spent
proofing the final manuscript.

CONTENTS

PREFACE

Touch has been described as the language of love. Along with the spoken word, body language, and eye contact, the act of touching, mediated through millions of tiny neurologic receptors in our skin, allows us to share the complex nuances and subtleties of our feelings with others.

Kissing, hand-holding, and stroking are just some of the diverse ways we use our skin to communicate. But whatever may be said about skin contact as a vehicle for communication for adults, it is especially true for infants and small children. Their primary experiences with the outside world are transmitted and interpreted through their skin. Scientists call touch *tactile contact*. The touch of a mother's hands and the feel of her body impart to newborns an essential, unspoken knowledge of the environment that becomes the foundation for their emotional reassurance within the awesome, incomprehensible world around them.

It has long been known that depriving newborns of touch can result in retarded psychosocial development and a failure to thrive (the inability to gain weight and grow properly). The noted anthropologist Ashley Montagu observed, "The more we learn about the effects of cutaneous stimulation, the more significant for healthy development we find it to be." Frederick Leboyer, the famed French obstetrician and developer of the natural childbirth technique that bears his name, went so far as to assert that touching, caressing, and massaging should be considered as "food for the infant." And this philosophy has found its way into the textbooks. One standard pediatric text states that the seemingly routine and automatic acts of "cuddling, rocking, bathing, and anointing the newborn infant" are essential for emotional and physical health. Clearly, then, anything that significantly interferes with tactile contact may have profound effects on a baby's overall health, well-being, and development. Put closer to home, if your baby's skin becomes sore, inflamed, or infected, his or her perception of the world is threatened with distortion. When this happens, the baby's previously secure environment can suddenly become more frustrating, hostile, and painful.

Few children are lucky enough to pass through infancy and early childhood without some skin problems. Some may arise suddenly, some may appear disfiguring, and all, especially to the new parent, may be baffling. Fortunately (for both you and your child), most common infant and early childhood skin conditions, regardless of how alarming they may appear, are temporary, nonscarring, and easily manageable through simple medical measures. Still, you need to be prepared to recognize problems early and to know what you can do for the simple ones and when to seek help in dealing with those that are more complicated. More than your child's physician, you play the key role in keeping your child's skin healthy and attractive.

It is here that *Baby Skin* can prove most helpful. It is intended as a handbook to answer the kinds of questions that anxious parents most frequently ask their child's pediatrician or dermatologist about a wide variety of skin subjects. The goals are to demystify problems and provide clear answers and explanations about what you can do for your child and what your doctor can do. I have made a great effort to translate confusing medical jargon into plain English.

Starting with the basics of proper infant and childhood skin care, the first two chapters cover subjects such as choosing the best soaps, cleansers, shampoos, laundry detergents, and moisturizers for your child's delicate skin; deciding between cloth diapers and regular or ultra disposables; the pros and cons of powders and lotions for diaper changes; and adequate sun protection. Subsequent chapters cover a wide range of common eruptions and conditions, such as worrisome-looking growths and spots, diaper rashes, insect bites, infections, special hair and nail conditions, blood vessel birthmarks, and a number of serious (and occasionally life-threatening) skin diseases. The book concludes with the various effects infants can have on the mother's or parent's skin, including pregnancy-related changes, nipple irritations from nursing, and hand eczemas.

Although the material in *Baby Skin* is in no way intended to substitute for appropriate medical consultation, it is offered in the hope of providing the necessary background to make you a more knowledgeable parent and a more confident participant in all aspects of your child's skin care. Given the nature of the book, however, the descriptions and explanations of medical therapies and surgical procedures must be addressed to the general concerns of a wide audience. If you have particular concerns about any form of therapy described here, you should, of course, ask your child's doctor.

Throughout *Baby Skin,* I have mentioned by brand name a variety of cosmetics and drugs for various conditions. These products are ones with which I have had considerable personal experience and have found consistently effective. I am not, however, endorsing any product or products or any generic substance. In most cases, the products cited are by no means the only ones available for dealing with the conditions discussed, nor does exclusion from my mention imply that a particular product is not equally effective. When products have been found worthless, I clearly say so. I do suggest, however, that you consult your dermatologist or pediatrician if you have any questions about the value or efficacy of a specific drug or cosmetic.

In sum, when a child's skin is normal and healthy, much love and enjoyment can be expressed between parent and child through touch. Ordinary child care duties, such as handling, feeding, bathing, and diapering, may be viewed as more than onerous, obligatory chores; they are also means of caressing—acts through which parents may transmit to their child unspoken signals of love, support, and reassurance. The bonding that results when there are no stumbling blocks to this communication can lay the groundwork for the broader, more intimate relationships of the future. I can certainly attest to this, not only from my professional experience but on a more personal level, as the father of five children. If this book, by making proper infant and childhood skin care easier and more comprehensible to new parents, helps maintain that wondrous, almost magical communication between parent and small child, and replaces parental worry with greater confidence, its goals will have been amply realized.

PART ONE

BASIC CARE

1

BABYING THAT PRECIOUS SKIN

Because baby skin looks and feels so different from adult skin, you may be surprised to learn that the three basics of caring for your infant's skin parallel those of caring for your own. They are (1) proper cleansing, (2) appropriate moisturization, and (3) adequate sun protection. The first two basics are discussed in this chapter. I have chosen to devote a separate chapter to sun protection because of its great impact on the long-term health and beauty of your child's skin.

PROPER CLEANSING

Considering the soiling that infants do and all the dirt and grime that older children continually get themselves into, keeping your child clean may sometimes seem like an impossible task. At the same time, the new parent can find juggling that tiny, slippery, wriggly baby in a bath a scary experience. I remember the feeling well. Rest assured, however, that after the first few times, you will grow quite confident and skillful. A gentle but firm grip is all you need to reassure your baby and make bathtime a special chance for the touching and caressing that are so crucial for your baby's development.

Strong soap, a sturdy sponge, and hot water are all wrong for taking care of human skin—and especially bad for the skin of infants and toddlers. Their oil glands are less well developed than adults' and function poorly. Consequently, strong soaps and cleansers, which degrease the skin, are unnecessarily drying and irritating to babies and young children.

Soaps and cleansers contain *emulsifiers* or *surfactants*. These are chemicals that lock onto grease, grime, environmental pollutants, and so on and make them easily rinsable from the skin with plain water. Because water ordinarily repels oils and grease, without emulsifiers it would be difficult to clean ourselves adequately. But, because our oil secretions are by their very nature greasy, the trick for the cosmetic or pharmaceutical chemist is to formulate a cleanser that removes only the bad greases and grime, leaving the good natural oils behind. To date, no product accomplishes this task perfectly, although a number do an adequate job.

The Cleanser Marketplace

There are several basic groups of soaps and cleansers to choose from, all capable of cleaning your child's skin adequately. However, the choice is somewhat complicated; at present, the jury is still out on just how gentle cleansers must be for children's skin. Until we clearly determine how much more vulnerable children's skin is compared with our own, it would seem prudent to avoid strong cleansers and those with potentially irritating or allergenic additives.

Toilet soaps are essentially modern-day versions of the age-old fat and lye soap formulas. In general, I don't recommend them for babies. They tend to be strong and highly alkaline and consequently have the potential to irritate skin more than necessary. In addition, in hard water areas of the country, they leave sticky, scummy deposits on the skin and in sink basins. These soaps are better tolerated by adults with thicker, oilier skin.

Superfatted soaps, for all practical purposes, are toilet soaps to which various moisturizers, such as cold cream, lanolin, mineral oil, or cocoa butter, have been added to offset the drying tendency. As a result, they are generally less effective cleansers than toilet soaps, but they perform adequately for ordinary cleansing needs. *Transparent soaps* can be thought of as superfatted soaps to which glycerin has been added. Because glycerin has a tendency to draw water from the skin, these soaps may be too drying for small children.

Special soaps, those containing antiseptics, deodorants, abrasives, fragrances, or herbal additives, should be avoided unless specifically recommended by your pediatrician or dermatologist. In general, these products cleanse no more efficiently than other soaps, but they are more likely to be drying, irritating, and even allergenic. Furthermore, it is unlikely that their additives confer any benefits, because they are immediately rinsed off.

Soapless soaps are synthetic detergent cleansers that usually contain fatty acids derived from petroleum chemicals. Often referred to by their manufacturers as *bars* or *cakes* to distinguish them from plain toilet soaps, these products clean adequately and leave no scummy residue. Lowila Cake is an example of these products and a good choice when a gentle cleansing cake is recommended.

Liquid cleansers are still another major category. Store shelves are filled with a wide range of these products, from cleansing lotions to liquid soaps. *Cleansing lotions* are simply moisturizers intended to be applied and then wiped off with a tissue. These products may not clean well enough. *Liquid soaps,* as their name suggests, are true soaps in liquid form, to which glycerin is sometimes added. These may be too harsh for a child's skin.

In between these extremes are two other types of liquid cleansers: washable lotions and sensitive skin cleansers. *Washable lotions* are cleansing lotions to which soap or detergent has been added.

Many baby bath products fit into this category. *Sensitive skin cleansers* are the liquid counterparts of the synthetic detergent cakes described earlier. Moisture sensitive skin cleanser is a gentle, fragrance-free liquid cleanser recommended for infant use.

The Best Routines

Before your baby can crawl, dirt on his or her skin essentially consists of drooled saliva and milk, "spit-up" around the mouth, chin, cheeks, and neck, perspiration, lint, and fecal and urinary soilage. For this delicate stage in your baby's life, tepid water baths are more than adequate. (Remember, hot water is too irritating.) If necessary, you can use a tiny amount of a liquid sensitive skin cleanser. Minimal rubbing, preferably with your fingertips, is best. You should avoid polyester scrub sponges, and even washcloths. Bathing every other day is more than enough for most infants.

The salts and enzymes in diaper waste can be particularly irritating to your baby's skin. Cleansing the diaper area with each change is therefore a must. Because fecal material can be especially adherent, you might find alcohol-free, fragrance-free wipes, such as Johnson's Baby Wash Cloths, particularly helpful. They are also convenient for travel and quite handy for older children, in place of toilet tissue, during toilet training. For a noninflamed diaper area, you can cleanse the skin with a soft cloth or cotton ball saturated with a hypoallergenic, paraben-free, lanolin-free, and fragrance-free moisturizer, such as Moisturel lotion. (See Chapter 6 for a discussion of diaper rashes and their treatments.)

Being the father of five boys, I know from personal experience just how dirty children can get once they become crawlers and toddlers. These are the stages when bars, cakes, or sensitive skin cleansers become essential.

Bubble Baths

Most preschoolers love to sit and play in baths, and bubble baths seem to be a particular attraction. Some children would stay in the bath for hours if you let them. Bubble bath products are detergent cleansers that contain ingredients capable of making water foamy. They are, nonetheless, soapy solutions that can irritate and overly degrease sensitive skin. For this reason, I do not recommend them. If you must use them, be sure to follow the manufacturer's instructions; overusage or overconcentration in the bath have been associated with severe skin and mucous membrane irritations, particularly of the urinary tract. If your child insists on frequent baths or enjoys lengthy bathtimes (or if you just enjoy the breather they give you), add a couple of capfuls of a bath oil product, such as Alpha Keri Oil, to your child's bath water. But make sure to use rubber bath mats, because water containing these products can become pretty slippery. Then sit back and relax.

Baby Shampoos

Much of what I said earlier about soaps can be said of shampoos. Despite what advertisers would like you to believe, shampoos are nothing more than cleansers for the hair. In other words, they should not be expected to do more than clean the hair of grease and oils. Baby shampoos are specifically formulated to be exceedingly mild, because the oil glands of babies and small children actually produce little oil. These shampoos contain *amphoteric* surfactants, emulsifiers that are nonstinging and nonirritating to the eyes—a giant plus when shampooing an often unwilling, if not loudly protesting, child.

Ordinary soaps and cleansers are too strong for children's hair and should be avoided. They can leave hair dull and lifeless looking. Even mild shampoos intended for adults with normal hair should be avoided, because they may contain stronger surfactants, such as sodium or ammonium lauryl sulfate, in higher concentrations than are needed. Finally, shampoos containing conditioning agents should also be avoided; these may contain proteins or herbal ingredients that are not only unnecessary but irritating.

Early on, your infant's hair may require only a gentle rinsing with plain, tepid water at bathtime. However, when your baby is older and more active, you will probably need to use a cleanser. A variety of baby bath and no-tears shampoos are available for this purpose. However, I prefer a fragrance-free product such as Moisturel sensitive skin cleanser, which may be used for both body and scalp. Whatever you choose, don't overdo it! Two to three times a week is about right, unless otherwise advised by your child's physician.

Doing the Laundry

As for soaps and shampoos, the rule for laundry products is to look for mild detergents—those containing as few potentially irritating or drying ingredients as possible. Cheerfree, a relative newcomer in the detergent market, though not specifically directed to the baby market, is perfume- and dye-free and my first choice. Or look for detergents marketed specifically for babies' laundry. It's a good idea to separate your baby's clothes from the rest of your wash, and avoid fabric softeners, and especially bleaches, whenever possible, not only on baby's clothes but on sheets, pillowcases, and so on. Special note: Ivory Snow in the powder form is a true soap, not a detergent, and is different from the liquid form. If you prefer the powder, you should also be aware that soaps may mask the flame-retardant capability of certain fabrics.

This is probably a good time for a few words about selecting clothing. Although normal skin can tolerate almost any type of clean outer garment, cotton and other loose-knit, natural fibers are generally more comfortable. By contrast, wool is more likely to tickle and barb the skin. Last, a newborn's heat-regulating, sweating mechanism is not yet fully developed; as a result, prickly heat reactions are more common when the skin becomes overheated. So, no matter what clothing you choose, dress your baby in layers and be sure not to overbundle.

APPROPRIATE MOISTURIZATION

In general, if you don't overbathe or oversoap your child, unlike for more mature skin, there should be little need for regular use of moisturizers. However, dry, chapping winds, dampness, indoor heating in winter, chlorine pools, oversunning (a no-no!), and air-conditioning in summer occasionally can dry out your child's skin. Under these conditions, a moisturizer can be helpful.

Moisturizers are big business. Over $650 million are spent annually on all-purpose moisturizers, and well over $1 billion more are spent on moisturizers for special body areas, such as the face and the hands. Ads for moisturizers can be as alluring as they are confusing. And with at least 350 all-purpose moisturizers available, choosing one without some guidelines can be confusing, to say the least.

Moisturizers range in price from several dollars for a few fluid ounces to well over a hundred dollars for half an ounce. Many contain additives, such as collagen, procollagen, elastin, vitamin E, vitamin A, herbal or cellular extracts, eggs, milk, honey, royal bee jelly, DNA, RNA, hyaluronic acid, liposomes, and allantoin, all of whose supposed health benefits remain unproven.

Advice on the subject recently offered by a leading consumer magazine still holds true: Spend more, get less! To save money, stick with an all-purpose moisturizer. You absolutely don't need one type for your child's face or hands and another for the rest of his body. And avoid those that contain any of the exotic-sounding ingredients just listed; they simply add to the cost and increase the risk of irritation. Also avoid those that contain fragrances, paraben preservatives, and lanolin or lanolin derivatives. These ingredients have been found to be irritating or allergenic for a goodly number of people. Finally, because the purpose of a moisturizer is not to add oils to the skin but to retain the skin's natural water, you should look for those that contain both *occlusive* ingredients (to lock in water), like petrolatum, and *humectants* (water grabbers), like glycerin. Moisturel lotion is an example of a relatively inexpensive, all-purpose, hypoallergenic moisturizer.

For best effect, lightly pat your child's skin dry after bathing. Do not vigorously towel. Follow immediately with an application of moisturizer, while the skin is still moist to wet rather than completely dry. In this way, moisture absorbed from the bath can be locked into the skin instead of lost to the atmosphere.

CHANGING DIAPERS

Although technically not part of the three basics of skin care, diapering makes up such a large part of child care during your child's first year or two that it deserves mention here. For a detailed discussion of diaper rashes, see Chapter 6.

These days, for convenience, 93 percent of American babies wear some form of disposable diapers. Nevertheless, the first question many mothers ask is which diaper is truly ideal: cloth, disposables, or the new ultras. That question is easy to answer. None. All three fail to meet the ideal of waste containment coupled with complete skin protection. However, of the three options, the ultras appear to be the most effective. Cloth diapers contain stool and urine through multiple layers of cotton supplemented by plastic overpants. By contrast, most disposable diapers consist of an absorbent core made from purified cellulose pulp, a plastic outer cover, and nonwoven fabric liner top sheet that contacts your baby's skin.

At their core, the newer ultras contain a polymeric (cross-linked polyacrylates) absorbent gelling material (AGM), which binds fluid and minimizes skin contact with moisture and irritants. Several recent studies have shown that ultras maintain skin dryness better than cloth diapers or conventional disposables and decrease both frequency and severity of diaper rashes. Acting as a buffering agent, the polymer in ultras also helps maintain the skin's normal, slightly acidic pH. The resulting decreased wetness has one drawback, however; parents often don't recognize when their baby has urinated.

Since *maceration,* or fragile skin resulting from overhydration, can pave the way for further irritation, ideally an infant's diaper should be changed immediately after each urination or bowel movement. In most cases, however, this ideal is seldom met. Newborns urinate on average at least twenty times per day and one-year-olds about seven times a day. According to recent surveys, most parents make only between five and ten diaper changes per day. Therefore, it would be reasonable to apply some additional protectant to the diaper area after each cleaning. Talcum powders, cornstarch, and various ointments all have their proponents.

Talcum powder is *ad*sorbent; that is, it repels water, keeping it from your baby's skin. It also reduces mechanical friction. *Cornstarch,* by contrast, is *ab*sorbent; it absorbs moisture, preventing it from coming into contact with the skin. It, too, reduces friction. I don't think there is sufficient evidence for one type of powder being better than another. In either case, however, I suggest that you avoid commercial baby powders and cornstarches because they generally contain fragrances. Inexpensive USP talc or plain household cornstarch will do very well, without the unnecessary scents. Apply sparingly before rediapering, and shield your baby's face when *patting* the powder on. A word of caution: Do not leave any powders in reach of your baby, and especially avoid those that come in nursing bottle–shaped containers. Serious injuries and even several deaths have resulted from infants sucking on these containers and breathing in and swallowing large volumes of powder.

If you prefer ointments or pastes, relatively inexpensive USP zinc oxide paste has been shown effective for minimizing wetness and irritation. Commercial products are no better, tend to be more expensive, and often contain potentially irritating additives.

2

THE PRIME DIRECTIVE: SUN PROTECTION

The sun is our skin's archenemy. Yet it seems that no matter how many times this message is repeated, it requires reemphasis. For young children in particular, adequate protection from the sun is vital as insurance against problems that could carry over into later years. Happily, by taking a few simple measures to prevent these problems, starting during your child's vulnerable infancy, you can do much to safeguard the present and future health of your child's skin and keep it looking smooth and radiant for years to come.

ADEQUATE SUN PROTECTION

Misconceptions about the supposed health benefits of sunning abound, and, although there really is no such thing, the notion of a "healthy tan" persists. Unfortunately, the nation's beaches remain crowded with sunbathers, and tanning parlors continue to proliferate.

By its very nature, a tan is the skin's response to ultraviolet damage. A little "color" means a little permanent damage; a deep tan means a lot of permanent damage. And a sunburn means even greater injury. In fact, *for each episode* of blistering sunburn during childhood and adolescence, an individual's lifetime risk of developing malignant melanoma doubles. All this bears witness to the need for stepped-up public education about the dangers of sun exposure and suntanning.

The overwhelming weight of medical and scientific evidence to date points to *ultraviolet* radiation from the sun (and from artificial sources, such as tanning parlors) as the culprit in 90 percent of the cosmetic damage to people's skin. A leathery or sallow complexion, "broken" blood vessels, sagging skin, and coarse or fine wrinkles are largely the results of accumulated sun damage.

At least 90 percent of skin malignancies are also attributable to ultraviolet radiation. Precancers and a variety of skin cancers, including a potentially lethal form, malignant melanoma, have all been linked to sun exposure. It is believed that nearly 80 percent of skin cancers hark back to sun damage before the age of eighteen. And although less is known about the precise effects of *infrared* radiation, the rays responsible for the sun's warming effects, there is some evidence that they also contribute to permanent skin damage.

Because there is generally a ten- to twenty-year lag between skin damage and the development of skin cancer, today's epidemic is the result of sun exposure in the 1960s and 1970s. At present, millions of Americans have been diagnosed with skin cancer, and to this pool 500,000 to 600,000 cases are added each year, according to the Skin Cancer Foundation, the National Cancer Institute, and the American Cancer Society. Approximately 40 percent of all newly diagnosed cancers are skin cancers, afflicting one in seven Americans. It is further reckoned that for each 1 percent drop in the ozone layer, we can expect a 2 percent rise in skin cancer statistics.

Of even greater concern, it has been estimated that malignant melanoma, which claims the lives of one-fifth of its victims within five years of diagnosis, will affect 1 out of every 135 white people this year and 1 out of every 90 by the year 2000. The incidence of this virulent disease has doubled since 1980 and continues to soar by nearly 4 percent a year worldwide. In the last decade alone, malignant melanoma has gone from being the third to the first most common malignancy in women between ages twenty-five and thirty.

Unfortunately, the skin is not the only target of the sun's rays. Constant bombardment by ultraviolet light can also damage the delicate lenses of the eyes. Just as it does to a piece of cellophane left by a window, ultraviolet light can turn a crystal-clear lens opaque and brownish. Eventually, cataracts and partial blindness may result. But that's not all; ultraviolet light, transmitted to the sensitive, pigmented retinal tissue at the back of our eyes, can also lead to ocular melanomas.

Children are at particular risk for these problems. For one thing, children's skin is more sensitive to ultraviolet damage; it is harmed more than adults' by equivalent amounts of radiation. For another, children have more time to play outdoors, and their activities are more likely to expose them to intense midday sun. The average child receives about three times as much UVB (the sunburn rays) exposure as the average adult. Finally, because previously damaged skin is known to be more vulnerable to further sun damage, skin that has been sun-injured early in life is at a disproportionate risk for harm later.

''BUNDLING UP'' FOR SUMMER

Doom and gloom aside, the good news is that today we can do a lot to protect our children from the sun's damaging rays. The American Academy of Dermatology, along with the cancer organizations mentioned on page 14, has clearly stated that we can *reduce* our children's lifetime likelihood of developing skin cancer by *78 percent,* just by following a few simple rules, especially during those critical first eighteen years of life.

The first and most important step for protecting infants and small children is to keep them out of the sun as much as possible. Sunshine from mid-April to mid-October is most intense between 11:00 A.M. and 3:00 P.M., so outdoor activities during these months should be planned for the early morning or late afternoon. A small infant should be taken out in a hooded carriage rather than an unshaded stroller. Dress your child in a broad-brimmed cotton sun hat, long pants, and a tightly woven, long-sleeved shirt. The hat should shield the ears and the back of the neck. For an older child, a relatively new product called Frogskins—a tight-weave, nylon "swimshirt"—may be useful. According to the manufacturer, the shirt, intended for wear in and out of the water, provides seven times the protection of an ordinary cotton T-shirt, or the equivalent of an SPF of 35 (see page 17).

Some words of caution: If you're at the seashore, do not be tempted to shade your baby under a boardwalk or a beach umbrella without additional sun protection. Nor should you be fooled by a partly cloudy day. Sixty to 80 percent of the sun's rays can be reflected off the sand and water onto your baby, just as nearly 80 percent of its harmful rays can pierce the cloud cover to deliver a nasty burn. The sun's invisible ultraviolet radiation can even penetrate a wet T-shirt and up to 3 feet of water.

MAKING THE RIGHT CHOICE

Sunscreens are not recommended for babies under six months of age. According to a recent FDA report, newborns may not yet possess the capability for metabolizing and excreting some of the chemicals in sunscreens that may be absorbed through the skin.

Some experts advise avoiding sunscreens for a child's entire first twelve months. For older children, however, there is no controversy. Sunscreens should be used regularly. Fortunately, despite the seemingly endless array of products available, choosing the proper sunscreen for your child does not have to be difficult.

SPF, or *sun protection factor,* numbers are the key. In general, the higher the number, the greater the protection. Put another way, if your child is very fair-skinned and would burn after only twenty minutes of unprotected sun exposure, using a product with an SPF of 15 would give him about 15 times twenty minutes (five hours) before he would burn. With an SPF of 30, it would take about ten hours. There are six skin types, ranging from skin that is fair and burns easily (Type 1) to black skin, which never burns (Type 6). Children with skin types 1 and 2 particularly should be diligently protected.

Since more than 7 percent of people may experience irritation from or an allergy to PABA (para-aminobenzoic acid), which is frequently found in sun protection products, I generally recommend PABA-free sunscreens. A water-fast sunscreen, in other words, a product that stays on well despite swimming or heavy perspiration, is also advisable. PreSun 29 For Kids is an SPF-29, PABA-free, water-fast sunscreen.

The lips need protection, too. They are particularly sensitive to the sun and need to be covered with a sunscreen-containing lip ice (PreSun, Chap Stick).

For any sunscreen to bind adequately to the skin, it must be applied in a dry, air-conditioned room, preferably fifteen to thirty minutes before going out. Apply to all exposed areas, and don't overlook the ears and back of the neck. Following brisk exercise, prolonged swimming, or vigorous towel drying, it would be wise to reapply your sunscreen. Further, because the actual protection your child will get is proportional to the amount of sunscreen you apply, you should slather it on, evenly and generously. As an example, if you put on only half the recommended amount of an SPF-15 sunscreen, your child may only get an approximate SPF of 7.

Two final points. There has been some concern lately that sunscreen use may actually increase the risk of skin cancer. Proponents of this theory argue that current sunscreens are largely effective for blocking UVB (the sunburn rays) while doing little against UVA rays. They maintain that, given a false sense of protection, sunscreen users will be encouraged to stay outdoors longer, risking considerable future harm from UVA. Few experts agree with this theory, though, because many available sunscreens actually do provide adequate UVA protection.

A second concern is that sunscreen use will interfere with vitamin D production, leading to a deficiency in this important substance, which is necessary for calcium metabolism. Although it is true that sunlight initiates vitamin D synthesis in the skin, it only requires a few minutes (not hours) to do so. And even that little bit of sun is unnecessary, thanks to the abundance of calcium and vitamin D–fortified foods found on our supermarket shelves. Diet can more than amply supply your child's vitamin D needs without entailing any risks from sun exposure.

THE ''EYES'' HAVE IT

Sun protection applies to your child's eyes as well. Although Americans spend almost $1 billion a year on sunglasses, visual comfort and style, rather than health considerations, usually dictate our choices. And neither high cost nor dark lenses necessarily guarantee adequate UV protection. In fact, contrary to conventional wisdom, some darker glasses may make things worse. By allowing the pupils to dilate, they may facilitate ultraviolet penetration to the eye's deeper structures.

Ideally, for maximal protection, sunglasses should absorb not only ultraviolet radiation but the blue bands of visible light, because there is some evidence that this light might also be harmful. Happily, there are some useful guidelines, analogous to SPF numbers, for choosing sun protective eyewear. The American National Standards Institute (ANSI) has set minimum standards for ultraviolet absorption; the notation Z-80.3, appearing on either the frame or the temple piece of a pair of sunglasses, means that the lenses meet or exceed acceptable standards. As a general rule, neutral gray or "smoked" tinted lenses absorb most ultraviolet radiation without creating too much color distortion. Naturally, sunglasses are only practical for older children, and shatterproof safety lenses are recommended.

Making It a Routine for Life

From the time your child is able to understand, he should be taught good sun protection habits, the same way he is taught other health and safety practices, such as brushing teeth and looking both ways when crossing the street. In the end, protecting your child's skin from its archenemy—the sun—is also cost-effective; using a sunscreen on the areas most at risk—the neck, face, and head—would only cost $3,000 over your child's entire lifetime, a small price to pay for ensuring lifelong skin health and enhanced attractiveness.

But education should not end in the home. Our schools must also get involved. Teachers should plan outdoor activities during those times of day when the sun's rays are least intense, and they should see to it that sunscreens are applied. In the classroom, children should be taught the risks of unprotected sun exposure the way they learn the hazards of cigarettes, alcohol, and drugs. The Task Force on Youth Education of the American Academy of Dermatology has created a curriculum for use in kindergarten through the third grade. "The ABCs for Fun in the Sun" is one part of this new and exciting package. For more information on how you can institute this curriculum in your schools, you may write to the Task Force on Youth Education, American Academy of Dermatology, P.O. Box 3116, Evanston, IL 60204-3116.

Pamphlets and materials on related subjects may also be obtained from the Skin Cancer Foundation, Box 561, New York, NY 10156, and the American Academy of Dermatology, 1567 Maple Avenue, Evanston, IL 60201, or through local chapters of the American Cancer Society and the National Cancer Institute.

PART TWO

SKIN PROBLEMS: DIAGNOSIS AND TREATMENT

3

COMMON MEDICAL TERMS AND PROCEDURES DEMYSTIFIED

A baby's skin may seem overly delicate, tender, and almost too fragile to touch. It might surprise you, therefore, to learn that a newborn's skin actually differs only slightly from that of an adult. These differences include being thinner, less hairy, less oil and sweat producing, and possessing looser links between cells. Nevertheless, you'll find it reassuring that undamaged skin in a full-term newborn is believed to be no more susceptible to irritation than its adult counterpart. Preemie skin, however, does appear to be more sensitive.

NORMAL SKIN

Your child's skin, just like yours, is not simply a lifeless sheet that holds the inner organs in place. It is a complex organ composed of three major layers, the epidermis, dermis, and subcutis, that serves many functions, some of which researchers have only recently begun to appreciate. Weighing 9 pounds in adults, the skin is by far the largest organ of the body, making up 15 percent of total body weight. At its thinnest point, it is $\frac{1}{150}$ inch thick and at its thickest $\frac{1}{4}$ inch. The uniqueness of the skin's components and architecture contributes to an almost amazing pliability and durability, which make possible its protective, stress-bearing, and mobility functions.

The uppermost, paper-thin layer of the *epidermis*, the *horny layer* or *stratum corneum*, is a sheet of flattened, nonliving cells that is shed and replaced approximately every two weeks. The major protein fiber composing this layer is *keratin*. Normally hydrated, the horny layer contains approximately 10 percent water. The major interface with our external environment, this important layer prevents the penetration of many substances that come into contact with the skin. It is also our first line of defense against the sun's harmful rays, blocking out approximately 10 percent of ultraviolet radiation.

The living, and much thicker *prickle cell layer*, or *stratum spinosum*, sits directly below and continually replenishes the horny layer. In addition, the cells in this layer secrete a variety of hormonelike substances, known as *growth factors*, which play a role in both immunity to infection and disease and the regulation of wound healing and repair, the skin's *homeostatic* (maintenance) functions. Investigators are only beginning to appreciate the wide-ranging effects of these chemicals.

The *basal cell layer* is the bottommost layer of the epidermis. Continuously reproducing and maturing, basal cells are responsible for supplying a new generation of cells for all the layers above, a process that normally takes about twenty-eight days. Octopus-shaped *melanocytes*, the pigment cells of the skin, are located here and there between the basal cells. Stimulated by sunlight, these specialized cells produce tiny melanin packages *(granules)* that are injected into the neighboring cells above. An excellent absorber of ultraviolet radiation, melanin is the skin's main natural defense against sunlight. It is interesting that, regardless of ethnic origin, all skin has the same number of melanocytes. Individual and racial variations in skin color are not the result of differences in the number of pigment-producing cells. Instead, racial variations reflect differences in the activity level of the melanocytes as well as the number and distribution of melanin granules. More simply, melanocytes are more active in darker skin than in lighter skin.

The *dermis*, the second major skin layer, houses a dense network of small arteries, veins, lymphatics, capillaries, and nerve endings (making the skin an exquisite organ for sensing pain, pressure, and temperature). Collagen and elastin fibers surround the tiny vessels and nerves and make up the bulk of the dermis. Collagen fibers give the skin its mechanical strength, and elastin, as its name suggests, its elasticity. Dermal blood vessels, branches of much larger vessels, supply nutrition and oxygen to the skin and remove metabolic wastes. Constriction and dilation of these vessels in response to heat and cold are responsible for maintaining our normal body temperature.

The *subcutis*, or fatty layer, by far the thickest layer of the skin, acts as the body's cushion against trauma and its reserve energy storage site. Hair follicles and three kinds of sweat glands are situated deep within the dermis or subcutis. *Eccrine* sweat glands, found all over the body, secrete a watery, colorless liquid whose evaporation from the skin surface helps cool us off. For this reason, they are by far the most important glands of the skin. *Sebaceous* glands (oil glands), most numerous on the face, scalp, upper chest, and back, secrete through the pores *sebum*, a waxy, fatty liquid that coats and moisturizes. Under hormonal influences, they usually begin secreting at puberty. The *apocrine* glands, the sweat glands involved in odor production, though present from birth, likewise do not mature and secrete until the onset of puberty. These glands

are in the armpits, groin, buttocks, and belly button region and
serve no known biological function.

Finally, a variety of cells, whose precise roles in regulating
immunity, allergy, and inflammation are just now being understood, are scattered through all layers of the skin. Some, such as
macrophages, lymphocytes, white blood cells, and *mast cells* are migrants,
which enter the skin from the dermal blood vessels. Others, called
Langerhans' cells, reside permanently in the skin. The specifics are
less important here than an overall appreciation of the complexity
of the skin and of just how vital it is to our general health. With
this understanding, proper care of your child's skin from early on
becomes not just an issue of present and future aesthetics but a
crucial matter of maintaining health.

DIAGNOSING AND TREATING
CHILDHOOD SKIN DISEASES

To establish a diagnosis and institute treatment, doctors generally
follow a prescribed set of steps. To be sure, this is an involved
process, but it can be made more comprehensible with a few
simple definitions and explanations. Your child's doctor will generally begin by taking a complete history of your child's condition
(essentially your story of exactly when and how things began and
progressed). This is followed by a complete examination of your
child's skin. At this point, the doctor usually has a fairly good idea
of the diagnosis, or at least the possibilities. For confirmation, the
doctor may then order special tests. And, once the diagnosis is
made, specific treatments, medications, or surgery are recommended. Finally, if necessary, additional tests may be ordered to
monitor your child's progress. Regardless of the specific condition,
the steps for investigating remain fundamentally the same.

The Look of Things Gone Wrong—Legions of Lesions

Although your child's skin is a highly complex organ, the specific ways it reacts to injury, infection, or inflammation are surprisingly limited. Skin specialists refer to these as *reaction patterns*, and a general familiarity with the more common types of reaction patterns is important for understanding more fully the various conditions, diseases, and treatments discussed in the following chapters. You might find it helpful to refer back to this chapter as you read through the book.

Skin abnormalities of any kind are usually referred to as *lesions*. And it is the size, number, and distribution of specific lesions that provide the physician with the necessary clues for making a precise diagnosis. Lesions take a variety of forms and generally carry descriptive names. Because these terms are referred to throughout the book, it would be worthwhile to familiarize yourself with them now. They are followed by a general discussion of the diagnosis and treatment of both common and serious skin conditions.

Cysts are liquid or gelatin-filled sacs. By appearance alone, they may be mistaken for nodules (see page 28). When touched, however, cysts, unlike nodules, impart a sensation of resilience, similar to the feel of pressing on a eyeball. Oil gland cysts, known as *sebaceous cysts,* are common examples.

Erosions are generally moist, oozing areas that result from the loss of a thin layer of overlying skin. The base of a broken friction blister is an excellent example. *Ulcers* are deeper and larger erosions, resulting from the loss of more overlying skin. *Crusts* result when dried blood, serum, or pus oozes from an open wound, sore, or ulcer. They may be thick or thin, easily removable or firmly adherent, and any mixture of yellow, green, red, and brown. The honey-colored crusts of the common childhood infection impetigo are examples.

Excoriations, despite their imposing name, are nothing more than ordinary scratch marks.

Fissures are painful, linear cracks in the skin near points of movement. They are frequently seen at the corners of the mouth where they may be caused by certain yeast infections or vitamin deficiencies.

Macules are perfectly flat areas of discoloration that can be of any size, shape, or color. Dilated blood vessels or freckles, which cause a reddish discoloration of the skin, are examples of macules. A *patch* is simply a large macule. Ordinary bruises and port wine stains are examples of patches.

Nodules are solid, roundish lesions that arise deep within the dermis or subcutis. A deep insect bite is one example. The term *tumor* is reserved for any benign or malignant skin lesion larger and deeper than a nodule.

Papules are small, solid, rounded bumps measuring less than ½ inch in diameter. They may be scaly, pointy, dome shaped, or flat topped. Ordinary moles, acne blemishes, warts, and skin tags are all examples of papules.

Papulovesicles are simply combination lesions, consisting of papules on which tiny blisters are found. Similarly, a *papulopustule* is a papule on which a tiny pustule sits.

Plaques are mesalike projections above the skin that are larger than ½ inch in diameter. Large, silvery-scaled plaques are typical of psoriasis.

Pustules are white, yellow, or greenish yellow, pus-filled papules. The "pus heads" of teenage acne are probably the best-known examples of pustules.

Scars result when lost or injured skin is replaced by new, dense fibrous protein. Scars can be either raised or sunken. Keloids and chicken pox scars are examples of both types. An *atrophy* is a depression that results from the abnormal thinning of one or all of the skin's layers.

Vesicles are tiny, clear or pale yellow, fluid-filled blisters measuring less than ¼ inch in diameter. Occasionally, they may be bloody. The herpes cold sore (fever blister) is a well-known example. *Bullae* (singular: *bulla*) are simply large vesicles.

Wheals are pale red or pinkish, round, oval, snakelike, or ring-shaped bumps that last no more than twenty-four hours in the same location. *Hives* are the most common example of wheals. The term *angioedema* is reserved for a swollen, deforming hive reaction.

How Things Shape Up

A diagnosis often rests on more than simply recognizing the kinds of lesions present. Your child's doctor must also consider their arrangement and distribution. Certain eruptions possess highly characteristic annular, bulls-eye, linear, or ringlike patterns. Others may be composed of numerous solitary lesions. Some eruptions may be confined to one area of the body, such as the back of the neck; others are widespread. Such differences can be critical. For example, finding tiny blisters grouped on or near the lip strongly suggests a herpes simplex (cold sore) infection. But finding such blisters scattered over the trunk and extremities would suggest chicken pox.

DIAGNOSTIC AND THERAPEUTIC PROCEDURES

Anesthetics

These days most dermatologic procedures are routinely performed in the doctor's office, using a topical or local anesthetic. Although reducing pain and anxiety is important for every patient, it is particularly so for young children.

The main advantage of *topical anesthetics,* those applied directly to the skin, is that no needles are required. Skin refrigerants, which work by temporarily freezing nerve endings until they are numb, may be used for very brief procedures. The doctor must work quickly, however, because their effects last only a few seconds. Fluro-Ethyl spray and ethyl chloride are the two most common skin refrigerants.

Relatively recently, a combination ointment known as EMLA, consisting of the anesthetics lidocaine and prilocaine, has been used successfully for more prolonged topical anesthesia. Applied to the skin under a patch that is left in place for between one and three hours before surgery, the ointment combination provides adequate anesthesia for minor procedures. Although it is being used in Europe, EMLA ointment is not yet commercially available in the United States.

For deeper and more prolonged local anesthesia, *injectable anesthetics* are required. The two most commonly used are Xylocaine (Lidocaine) and Novocain (procaine). Epinephrine (adrenaline), a blood vessel–constricting agent, is frequently combined with these anesthetics to prolong the anesthetic effect and reduce bleeding. In the hope of reducing some of the discomfort of the injection, a small amount of bicarbonate of soda is also sometimes added to lower the acidity of the solution. In many cases, the doctor will freeze the skin with a topical refrigerant or an ice cube before injecting the anesthetic and will use an ultrafine, silicone-coated needle. Anesthesia usually lasts between thirty and ninety minutes, depending on the anesthetic used.

General, inhalational, or *intravenous anesthesia* is seldom required for childhood skin surgery, except when large or complex procedures are contemplated. Occasionally, nitrous oxide, or laughing gas, may be used to supplement the local anesthetic. Procedures requiring general anesthesia are performed in a hospital operating room or in special outpatient settings designed for more extensive surgery and monitoring.

Biopsies

When the history and examination of your child's condition are not sufficient for a diagnosis, your doctor may suggest a skin biopsy. A *biopsy* is a minor surgical procedure in which a small piece of skin is removed, usually under local anesthesia, and sent to the pathology laboratory for microscopic analysis. Accurately diagnosing many skin conditions requires the combination of clinical and microscopic analyses.

Skin biopsies are generally named for the instrument or method used to obtain the tissue sample. For example, a *punch* biopsy is performed with a cookie cutter–like, stainless steel instrument that cores out a small sample. A *curette* biopsy is performed using a razor-sharp, looplike instrument with a long handle to scoop out the desired sample. An *incisional* biopsy employs the traditional surgeon's scalpel to cut out only a piece of some large lesion. By contrast, an *excisional* biopsy involves cutting out the entire specimen along with some of the surrounding normal skin. A *shave* biopsy, probably the most common type of skin biopsy performed, involves using a scalpel to "shave" or sculpt a tissue sample horizontally off the skin. Individual circumstances usually dictate which procedure your doctor will choose.

These same procedures may be used surgically to treat lesions when the diagnosis is known. And, once again, the procedure is named for the method of removal. When, for example, a curette is used to remove a growth, the procedure is called *curettage* (eliminating the word *biopsy* because the purpose of the procedure is treatment rather than diagnosis). Similarly, when the dermatologic surgeon uses a scalpel to remove a growth, the procedure is referred to as *excisional surgery* (again the word *biopsy* is dropped to denote treatment rather than diagnosis).

Dermabrasion

Dermabrasion, or "skin sanding," long used in the treatment of acne scarring and wrinkling in adults, has been gaining favor recently in removing selected types of large, congenital nevi in children (see page 156). After freezing the skin with a skin refrigerant, such as Fluro-Ethyl spray, to stiffen and numb it, several types of motor-driven brushes are used to finely "sand" away the surface layers of the skin. Following treatment, new skin usually grows in within a week, and complete healing generally takes about three weeks. No stitches are needed. While children often require preoperative sedation, supplemental local anesthesia is ordinarily unnecessary.

Electrosurgery

Electrosurgery is the umbrella term for surgical procedures using electricity. More specifically, *electrodesiccation* is when the skin surgeon uses a high-frequency, alternating electric current to dehydrate unwanted tissue. Two other electrosurgical techniques, *electrocoagulation* and *electrocautery* rely on the intense heat generated by an electric current to "boil" tissue. Electrosurgical procedures are generally performed under local anesthesia and require no stitches.

Chemical Applications

Caustic chemicals have been applied to "burn" away unwanted growths, such as warts, for decades. In general, the procedure stings only momentarily and usually does not require either topical or local anesthetics, an obvious advantage in dealing with children. Trichloroacetic acid (TCA) in varying concentrations is the agent most commonly applied, although others, such as phenol, may occasionally be used. After degreasing the skin with acetone, the doctor applies the acid with a cotton-tipped applicator; within seconds, there is a stinging and a whitening of the skin, at which time the acid is neutralized with alcohol or plain water. Over the next several days, the treated skin peels away and new skin forms.

Cryosurgery

Cryo- means "cold," and *cryosurgery* involves using a freezing material to destroy tissue (not to just numb it, as with topical refrigerants). Ice crystal formation within treated lesions is responsible for tissue destruction. Dry ice (solid carbon dioxide) and liquid nitrogen are the two most common freezing materials currently employed. Liquid nitrogen is applied with either a cotton-tipped applicator or a special spray device. The cold is so intense and so instantly numbing that local anesthesia is seldom required.

Radiation Therapy

Radiation therapy (radiotherapy, or *X-ray therapy)* is usually reserved for treatment of certain more serious conditions, such as skin cancers. Treatments, which last from a few seconds to a few minutes, are not uncomfortable (they're like getting a chest X ray), and, except in the most uncooperative children, require no sedation or anesthetics. In general, radiation therapy is not recommended for small children, because its "weathering" effects on the skin may become apparent ten to twenty years after treatment, when the individual is still quite young.

Mohs' Chemosurgery

Mohs' chemosurgery, or *Mohs' micrographic surgery,* is a highly specialized form of cancer surgery, usually reserved for recurrent growths or growths in areas where high rates of recurrence are known to follow conventional treatments. In this procedure, the entire growth is mapped; then portions of it are systematically sliced out and examined under a microscope for residual malignancy. The procedure is repeated until all the cancer has been removed. In general, no stitches are required. However, when a large amount of tissue is removed, skin grafts may be required to close the wound.

Lasers

Lasers are powerful beams of selected wavelengths of visible or near-visible light. Focused on unwanted tissue, lasers, which can be thought of as funnels of energy, cause tissue boiling and cellular explosion. Carbon dioxide, argon, and neodymium-YAG lasers are the most common in routine medical use today. Each device possesses a particular therapeutic usefulness.

Lasers have proven their worth in several areas of medicine, including retinal and urologic surgery. In dermatology, lasers, particularly the carbon dioxide laser, are used to treat a variety of growths, such as warts and small tumors. Nevertheless, controversy still exists about their overall value compared with the simpler, often less expensive methods previously described. In the treatment of port wine stains, however, lasers have clearly demonstrated their superiority over any other method (see Chapter 12).

Topical, Intralesional, and Systemic Medications

Fortunately, physicians today have at their disposal an extensive array of medications to treat or cure many skin diseases. Specific therapies for individual conditions are discussed in the appropriate sections of this book. However, for a more complete understanding, some common medical terms need to be defined.

A *topical medication* is any drug applied to the skin that in some way affects the skin's structure and function. By contrast, a *cosmetic* is something applied to the skin merely to beautify and enhance it. Pure cosmetics, therefore, are not topical drugs, and any claim by a cosmetic to be "therapeutic" is misleading.

Topical medications can be formulated in cream, lotion, gel, ointment, powder, or spray vehicles. A *vehicle* is simply the preparation into which the active ingredient is placed.

Creams are by far the most commonly used vehicles in dermatology. Basically, they are fat, oil, and water blended to form a vanishing base. And, depending on the particular need, creams may be made more oily or more watery in consistency.

Lotions are essentially creams to which more water has been added to enhance spreadability. They can more easily be applied to hairy areas without causing much matting. Shake lotions, like the familiar calamine lotion, are nothing more than suspensions of various powdery substances in a lotion base.

Ointments are greasy vehicles, consisting of animal or vegetable fats or synthetic oily substances, such as cetyl and stearyl alcohols, and polyethylene glycol. The sticky, tacky feeling of many ointments limits their desirability. However, they are quite lubricating and have the additional advantage of promoting absorption of their active ingredients.

Gels are nonoily mixtures of water and alcohol. Liquefying on contact with the skin, they are useful for delivering a variety of active ingredients. On the down side, they sometimes cause stinging and excessive dryness.

Powders are pulverized materials excellent for drying and reducing friction. At the same time, they make an uneconomical and inefficient way to deliver other medications to the skin. They should be gently patted on, rather than dusted, to reduce chances of inhalation. *Pastes* are mixtures of powders and ointments.

Sprays, or aerosols, the last type of topical vehicle, have no place in the care of childhood skin problems. They are drying and deliver active ingredients inefficiently, and special caution must be exercised to prevent them from getting in the eyes.

Intralesional injections are therapeutic shots instilled directly into the abnormal tissue. Discomfort is the obvious disadvantage of any injection. The main advantage is that a small but concentrated amount of drug can be administered right where it is needed without exposing the entire body to its effects.

Finally, *systemic medications,* as their name implies, are drugs that enter the general system. These may be administered *orally,* which means they enter the bloodstream after they are broken down in the digestive system. They may be injected *intramuscularly,* which means they are slowly drawn from the muscle into the circulatory system, or *intravenously,* directly into the veins. Systemic therapies, particularly systemic steroid or antibiotic treatments, are often used to treat more severe skin conditions (see Chapters 7, 8, and 9).

This chapter is not intended to turn you into a dermatologist. Being able to diagnose and treat skin diseases takes not only a traditional medical school education but at least four years of additional training in both medical and surgical aspects of skin diseases, coupled with a lot of practice and experience. Nonetheless, familiarizing yourself with the fundamentals given here, and referring back to them as you read through this book, will prove invaluable.

4

NOT EVERY RASH IS A CATASTROPHE

Babies get rashes. It's a fact of life. And skin problems, either directly or indirectly, are responsible for about 30 percent of all childhood visits to the doctor. Although many rashes are scary looking, they are not necessarily serious or permanently harmful in any way. Many are nothing more than temporary nuisances that can be easily and effectively treated. This chapter, though not exhaustive, discusses the most common nonserious skin eruptions that can occur during the first months of your baby's life.

PEELING SKIN

Newborn skin is ordinarily covered by a greasy, grayish white, membranelike substance known as the *vernix caseosa,* composed of oil gland secretions and dead surface skin cells. The precise function of the vernix is still not understood, although it is believed to be somehow protective. Because it flakes and scales away during the first few weeks of a baby's life, the vernix is sometimes mistaken for a rash. Although it is ordinarily cleansed from the face in the nursery, it should be left to peel off on its own elsewhere on the body with washing and changes of clothing.

Vernix peeling often coincides with normal *(physiologic)* shedding of the skin, which usually begins within one to two days after delivery. This process, referred to as *desquamation,* may continue for two weeks. Assuming there are no other problems, once all peeling, flaking, and shedding is complete, your baby's skin will take on a soft, smooth, and velvety appearance.

SUCKING BLISTERS

Believe it or not, babies suck inside the womb. As a result, oval blisters, caused by the mechanical irritation of sucking, are commonly found at birth. Usually only one blister appears, typically on the hand, wrist, or forearm. However, multiple sucking blisters have also been found on both hands, and even on the feet. These blisters are harmless and disappear completely as soon as your baby begins the preferred substitutes of breast or bottle feeding. Diagnosis of sucking blisters is usually easy, although your doctor may occasionally need to exclude other causes of blistering in the newborn.

ACROCYANOSIS

Shortly after birth, the skin, particularly on the arms and legs, is normally purplish red. Soon thereafter it changes to pink, although this change occurs more slowly on the lips, hands, and feet. In many infants, however, cold temperatures, crying, and breath-holding spells may provoke a temporary but marked constriction of the blood vessels in the lips, hands, and feet, deepening the discoloration. This perfectly normal reaction is known as *acrocyano-*

sis. The transient nature of the discoloration, and the absence of other symptoms, helps your doctor distinguish this problem from true *cyanosis,* a condition in which heart or lung problems lead to poor oxygenation of the blood and a permanent bluish-purpling of the entire skin.

CUTIS MARMORATA (MARBLED SKIN)

Cutis marmorata, or *marbled skin,* is another innocuous and transient blood vessel abnormality common after birth. It generally appears following a drop in temperature. In this condition, the newborn's blood vessels are superficial and dilated and show up prominently on the surface of the skin. The term *marbled skin* reflects the similarity between these striking blood vessel configurations on the skin and the characteristic patterns of veined marble. Cutis marmorata is so common that it is considered normal. It disappears without treatment.

HARLEQUIN COLOR CHANGE

Used here, the term *harlequin* means bright and parti-colored, like the dress of a clown. In *harlequin color change,* when the baby lies on his side, the side of the body against the mattress reddens while the opposite side blanches. A striking line of demarcation separates the two halves. In milder forms, the demarcation is less pronounced; the genital region and certain areas of the face may not be involved. Attacks may last from a few seconds to as long as thirty minutes.

Harlequin color change is found more frequently in premature infants. However, it is also seen in as many as 10 percent of normal, full-term deliveries. Starting within a few days of birth, the condition may continue for two to three weeks. Like cutis marmorata, harlequin color change, though striking, is entirely harmless to the baby. It is believed to be related to a temporary lag in maturation of the lower brain center that controls blood vessel dilation and contraction. A thorough pediatric examination is strongly suggested, though, if a baby has this condition, because some cases of harlequin color change have been linked with brain injury.

SALMON PATCHES

Salmon patches are by far the most common neonatal blood vessel abnormality, occurring in as many as 40 percent of newborns. Also known as *telangiectatic nevi* or *nevi simplex,* these dull, flat, pinkish or salmon-colored spots represent dilated capillary remnants of fetal circulation that are yet to be replaced by more mature capillaries. Salmon patches are most commonly found on the nape of the neck, but symmetrical involvement of both eyelids is also quite common. They are also frequently located along the midline of the face—on the forehead, between the eyes, and on the upper lip. Salmon patches are often referred to by such fanciful names as *stork bite* when on the nape of the neck and *angel's kiss* when between the eyes.

As a rule, salmon patches are perfectly harmless. In 95 percent of cases, they disappear before the infant's first birthday leaving no residual skin discoloration, although approximately 50 percent of those found on the nape of the neck persist lifelong. In these cases, because the back of the neck will usually be covered by hair as the child grows older, the condition can simply be ignored. It is interesting that long after the spots fade, crying, breath holding, or vigorous exercise may trigger a slight reddening of a previously affected site, especially in very fair-skinned children.

Other developmental blood vessel problems and their treatments are discussed in Chapter 12.

TRAUMATIC PURPURA

Despite the best prenatal and obstetrical care, a baby's entrance into this world is sometimes fraught with mishap. *Purpura*, which means "bruising or bleeding (hemorrhage) into the skin," can result from rough travel through the birth canal or from a complication of a difficult delivery. Examples include prolonged spontaneous deliveries, which permit considerable molding of the head, or forceps deliveries that result in swelling and bruising. Though often frightening in appearance, most such swelling and bruising is harmless, resolving spontaneously in days to weeks without any scarring or permanent damage.

TOXIC ERYTHEMA (ERYTHEMA TOXICUM NEONATORUM)

Despite the word *toxic* in its name, this very common rash is a completely harmless condition. Its precise cause remains unknown, although there is speculation that it may be a temporary, atypical reaction to ordinary stimuli like heat or mechanical irritation. *Toxic erythema* affects about half of all full-term newborns and, to a much lesser extent, preemies.

Ordinarily beginning in the first two days of a baby's life, the rash initially appears as flat, irregular, splotchy, reddish lesions, usually on the trunk. Soon after, tiny papules and pustules form within the reddish blotches; the rash may then progress to virtually any other skin area, sparing only the palms of the hands and soles of the feet. In mild cases, very few lesions are seen; in more widespread instances, literally hundreds may develop. Because of the presence of various combinations and stages of papules and pustules astride reddish bases, toxic erythema is often referred to as the flea-bitten rash of the newborn.

Toxic erythema requires no treatment and usually disappears

spontaneously in approximately ten days. Periods of worsening and calming are typical during this time. Occasionally, your child's doctor may need to order special tests to help distinguish this eruption from certain bacterial conditions or widespread herpes infection (see Chapter 9), a much more serious, and potentially life-threatening, condition.

CRADLE CAP

Cradle cap is a scaly, crusty, cracking scalp rash, which is most common during the first two to twelve weeks of infancy. It is believed to be one manifestation of seborrheic dermatitis, a condition that may also affect the face, diaper region, and body fold areas (see Chapter 7). Cradle cap is the counterpart of ordinary dandruff, or seborrhea. Sometimes dry and whitish, the scales are more typically red-orange, greasy looking, and sticky. The precise cause of cradle cap is unknown, although there is indirect evidence linking it to stimulation by maternal hormones transferred across the placenta before birth.

Cradle cap generally does not itch and usually clears by age one. In most cases, no special therapy is needed, just routine, gentle cleansing and shampooing to remove scales and debris. In tougher cases, the occasional use of Capitrol, or an antidandruff sulfur- and salicylic acid–containing shampoo such as Sebulex, can be useful. In persistent cases, your doctor may prescribe a mild topical corticosteroid lotion, such as Hytone.

TRANSIENT NEONATAL PUSTULAR MELANOSIS

This tongue twister is the name of a harmless condition seen most commonly in black infants. The rash of *transient neonatal pustular melanosis,* which may be present at birth, starts as small vesicopustules, usually on the forehead, neck, chin, lower back, and shins. In some infants, only a few lesions appear, whereas in others, numerous clusters develop everywhere, including on the palms of the hands and soles of the feet. Within twenty-four hours of appearance, each blister-pustule breaks down, leaving a circular scale (known as a collarette) surrounding a flat, pinhead-sized, brownish stain. The cause of the eruption is unknown.

Outbreaks may persist for from several weeks to months. And the brownish stains generally require between three weeks and three months to fade completely. No treatment is necessary. When the diagnosis is less certain, your child's doctor may consider additional tests to exclude bacterial, viral, yeast, or parasitic infections that can mimic this condition.

INFANTILE ACROPUSTULOSIS

The harmless rash of *infantile acropustulosis*, which usually begins in children somewhere between two and ten months of age, consists of recurrent episodes of intensely itchy pustules or pustular blisters, mainly on the hands and feet. The palms and soles are favored locations. Initially, breakouts can occur as often as every two weeks; later they may recur at intervals of several weeks. The problem generally clears spontaneously by around the second or third birthday. Your child's doctor may prescribe something for the itch.

MILIARIA RUBRA (PRICKLY HEAT)

The very common rash *miliaria rubra* (or *prickly heat*) occurs when there is clogging of the eccrine sweat ducts (see Chapter 3); sweat retention and the release of highly irritating sweat *under the skin* are believed to trigger the eruption. Typical lesions of miliaria are reddish papules or papulovesicles, and the forehead, trunk, neck, armpits, and groin are the most common sites of involvement. Premature infants with incompletely developed sweat apparatus are particularly susceptible, although virtually all children can develop this condition under the right environmental conditions.

Named for the prickling sensation it causes, miliaria is harmless. Lower room temperature and humidity, cool baths, and loose, lightweight clothing usually constitute the only treatment necessary. Powders can also be helpful.

Prickly heat has several variants. *Miliaria crystallina* (also called *sudamina*) develops when the sweat ducts are clogged high in the horny layer of the skin. The clear, tiny, thin-roofed vesicles characteristic of this related condition may develop after excessive sweating caused by high temperature or humidity, after sunburn, or in response to a fever. As in ordinary prickly heat, the scalp, trunk, armpits, and groin are most often affected. Itching, however, is not a problem.

Miliaria pustulosa, another relative of prickly heat, is believed to be simply a progression of miliaria rubra. Here, pustular lesions develop in addition to the typical rash. Prolonged sweat duct clogging, increased amounts of trapped sweat, and more inflammation are believed to be responsible for this reaction. Once again, treatment must be directed to dressing the baby in looser clothing and lowering room temperature and humidity. When the diagnosis is less certain, your child's doctor may order cultures to eliminate the possibility of a bacterial infection.

NEONATAL ACNE

Believe it or not, acne, the dread of adolescence, is quite common in newborns and infants. Outbreaks of *neonatal acne,* like those of teenage acne, typically consist of pimples and pustules primarily on the cheeks, chin, and forehead. In contrast to adolescent acne, in newborn acne the chest and back are spared. Neonatal acne is more common in boys than girls and is believed to result from male hormone stimulation of sebaceous glands that have not yet shrunk to their childhood state of immaturity.

Neonatal acne generally clears by itself during the first few months of life. Other than routine daily cleansing, treatment is rarely needed. In more persistent cases, a mild keratolytic, for instance, Rezamid lotion, may be tried, or a benzoyl peroxide–containing agent, such as Desquam-E 2.5 emollient gel, may be prescribed.

INFANTILE ACNE

Infantile acne, which can begin when a child is about three or four months of age, is a more serious form of neonatal acne, consisting of whiteheads, blackheads, pimples, pustules, and even potentially scarring cystic lesions. The course of this condition varies. Milder cases may abate spontaneously in a few weeks. Most cases, however, take one to two years to disappear. A few cases have been reported to persist into puberty. Once again, therapy is determined by severity. Milder cases require only routine daily cleansing. More severe cases can benefit from the prescription medications used for teenage acne.

Children with this problem who have a strong family background of acne are felt to be at particular risk for severe outbreaks during adolescence. To prevent complications, after puberty these children should be monitored closely by a dermatologist, and they should be treated as early as possible.

5

ODD-LOOKING GROWTHS AND SPOTS YOU DON'T HAVE TO WORRY ABOUT

Just as not every rash on your child is a catastrophe, not every spot, bump, or growth is a calamity. Even many so-called developmental abnormalities—atypical conditions arising in the course of your child's development—are perfectly innocuous. Many require no more therapy than the doctor's reassurance.

BREAST SWELLING

Breast swelling is not uncommon immediately after birth and is believed to be related to the passage of certain nursing-related maternal hormones across the placenta during pregnancy. Occasionally, even milk spillage occurs. This condition can be seen in infant boys as well as girls.

Although it may persist for some time after birth, breast swelling is of no consequence and will disappear spontaneously. Under no circumstances should you attempt to massage or milk the breasts. This may not only irritate them but lead to infection.

SUPERNUMERARY APPENDAGES

Supernumerary is a mouthful, but the term simply means "more than a normal number." An individual with *supernumerary nipples*, therefore, was born with more than the usual two. To accommodate large litters, many mammals, such as dogs and cats, possess milk lines, rows of breasts that extend from the chest area to the pubic area on both sides. In humans, the potential for developing multiple breast tissue sites is apparently retained.

Supernumerary nipples are surprisingly common in both sexes. Infant girls may even develop full glandular breast tissue along the entire length of the milk lines on both sides, although this occurs only occasionally in males. In most cases, the diagnosis is obvious, but supernumerary nipples are occasionally mistaken for ordinary moles. In either sex, the condition is perfectly harmless, and simple excision of the excess tissue is curative.

Auricular tags, another fairly common form of supernumerary appendages, are fleshy outcroppings around the ears. In general, they appear as flesh-colored nubs of tissue, which may be confused with moles or ordinary papillomas. Simple shave excision followed by electrosurgical cautery (see Chapter 3) of the base of each lesion is curative.

Auricular tags sometimes contain cartilage or are linked to deeper, vital structures in the external canal or middle ear. In such cases, more extensive and delicate surgery is required.

NEVUS ANEMICUS

The word *nevus* is frequently used loosely to refer to ordinary pigment spots or moles, also called *beauty marks* and *birthmarks*. More precisely, however, *nevus* refers to any spot or growth, especially one that is odd or abnormal, that results from inheritance or faulty embryologic development. It is in this broader sense that *nevus* is used here.

Nevus anemicus, a round or oval patch of pale or mottled skin, may be present at birth or develop in early childhood. The condition is harmless and is believed to represent an abnormally diminished ability of the small blood vessels to dilate properly when stimulated. It can also result from oversensitivity of these vessels to natural blood vessel–constricting hormones. Nevus anemicus commonly involves the chest and back. A quick test, rubbing a patch briskly, highlights the spot; the surrounding area reddens, while the spot remains unchanged in color. No effective therapy, other than cover-up cosmetics, exists. Covermark, Esteem, and Dermablend are three brands of specially formulated, water-fast masking makeups (see page 149).

NEVUS ACHROMICUS

Also known as *nevus depigmentosus, nevus achromicus* is nothing more than a pale patch on the skin, usually present at birth. Frequently linear or band shaped, these lesions may be quite small or cover larges areas of the body. Their pale color has been attributed to a reduced number of properly functioning pigment cells (melanocytes) and to melanin deficiency. If desired, a cover-up cosmetic is the only therapy needed.

MILIA

Located just below the skin surface, *milia,* which closely resemble whiteheads, are tiny sebaceous cysts packed with trapped cellular debris and oil gland secretions and lacking openings to the surface. Found in nearly 50 percent of infants, they typically appear as pencil-point-sized, pearly white or yellow papules on the forehead, nose, and cheeks. Occasionally, they develop on the upper trunk, limbs, penis, and even in the mouth.

Milia are perfectly harmless and usually disappear spontaneously by the time the infant is three or four weeks old. Rarely, they persist for two or three months. Although no treatment is necessary, if you wish, your child's doctor can remove them by nicking their surfaces with a fine needle or scalpel and expressing the contents. Milia treated in this fashion seldom recur.

OVERGROWN OIL GLANDS (SEBACEOUS GLAND HYPERPLASIA)

Maternal hormones, which linger in your baby's system after birth, can also stimulate the sebaceous glands, resulting in a condition known as *sebaceous gland hyperplasia,* or what I've termed *overgrown oil glands.* One or more of these bumps, which are usually small and yellow, orange-yellow, or flesh colored, may be found on the nose, cheeks, and upper lips. The problem is temporary and usually resolves spontaneously within the first few weeks of life, as the infant's maternal hormone levels fall. No treatment is needed.

EPIDERMAL NEVI

Arising entirely within the epidermis, as their name indicates, *epidermal nevi* are warty or thickened bumps on the skin. They vary from flesh color to deep brown and may assume round, oval, or even linelike shapes. One or more epidermal nevi may develop, each usually no larger than an inch in diameter. Most often, they are present at birth; less commonly, these nevi develop during infancy and rarely during later childhood.

Nevus unius lateris is a special type of epidermal nevus, noteworthy for its size and elaborate patterns. It may be a solitary, linear growth that courses down an entire limb in featherlike and marbled patterns, or galaxylike whorls that appear on more than half of the body. The scalp, face, and neck are frequently involved when such extensive patterns occur.

Despite the extent of their involvement, epidermal nevi are harmless and seldom become malignant. Cosmetic considerations are therefore the main reason for treatment. As with almost any growth of this kind, the procedure your doctor selects will depend on the age of the child and, most important, the location and extent of the problem. Scalpel removal, dermabrasion, electrosurgery, and cryosurgery have all been used with varying degrees of success. Unfortunately, regardless of the procedure, recurrences necessitating retreatment are common. Finally, because certain skeletal, neurologic, and heart abnormalities have occasionally been associated with the more extensive epidermal nevi, a thorough pediatric examination is advisable.

PIGMENTED SPOTS AND GROWTHS

Happily, most pigmented spots and growths have no effect on your child's overall health and development. For most individuals, they are nothing more than cosmetic nuisances. To others, they become so highly prized that they are referred to as *beauty marks*. The following sections describe the most common kinds of pigmented lesions found in infants and small children.

Nevi

Pigmented moles are the most common growths in humans and may appear almost anywhere on the body, including the mouth, anus, and genitals. They are found in 1 to 3 percent of newborn whites and upward of 16 percent of newborn blacks. Varying widely in appearance, moles assume three basic shapes: flat, slightly elevated, and dome shaped.

Moles that are perfectly flat, called *junctional nevi* (singular: *nevus*), range in color from light to dark brown and are ordinarily hairless. Although some may be oval or elliptical, most junctional moles are round and evenly colored. If you close your eyes and run your fingers across their surface, you should not be able to feel them. Junctional nevi are so called because the special cells composing them are located just above the junction between the dermis and the epidermis.

Flat moles are common in children and are believed to represent a first phase in the development of the raised moles of adolescence and adulthood. It is interesting that moles on the palms of the hands and soles of the feet do not progress and remain flat throughout life.

Moles that are slightly elevated, called *compound nevi*, are more common in older children, although they are occasionally seen in infants. Except for being elevated, they differ little in appearance from their flat counterparts. Some, however, can have a rough, warty-looking surface, and others, particularly those on the face, may have dark, coarse hairs growing out of them that become thicker and darker when the child reaches puberty. (Contrary to a popular myth, hairs within a mole do not make it more likely to be or turn malignant.)

Dome-shaped moles, or *intradermal nevi,* are much more common in adults, but children may get them, too. Sometimes flesh colored, they may be any shade of brown and are typically located on the head or neck. Coarse hairs may also be present. These nevi, which may vary in size from the width of a dime to more than ½ inch in diameter, may be either broadly attached to the surrounding skin or suspended by a narrow stalk. It is interesting that, by a person's thirties and forties, the pigment cells in moles are often replaced by fibrous or fatty tissue, so that few older people have any remaining moles.

Regardless of its appearance, should any mole change in size, shape, or color, you should have your child's dermatologist confirm that the change is merely a part of normal development. When a malignancy is suspected, a biopsy is usually performed.

Aesthetic considerations are the only reason for removing benign moles. Depending on its precise shape and location, an unwanted mole may be removed by shave or scalpel excision (see Chapter 3), usually with excellent cosmetic results. Of the two, I prefer the shave method, because it removes the mole flush with the surrounding skin surface and no stitches are needed. Although understandably disturbing to both parent and child, recurrence of the mole after removal in no way signals malignancy.

Nevus Spilus

Nevus spilus is a flat, nonhairy, pale brown patch speckled by numerous smaller, dark brown spots. Basically, this benign, fairly common lesion is a variation of the types of nevi just described. Lesions range from approximately ½ inch to 10 inches in diameter, with the face, trunk, and extremities being favored locations. Reassurance that the condition is benign is all the therapy necessary.

Halo Nevus

A *halo nevus* is a unique type of mole because it is surrounded by a patch of otherwise normal but depigmented skin. The central nevus may be junctional, dermal, or intradermal. The surrounding halo may vary from about ⅛ inch to as much as ½ inch in diameter. Although the trunk is the most common site of occurrence, halo nevi may develop anywhere on the body except the palms of the hands and soles of the feet, nail beds, and mucous membranes. Although they typically appear during adolescence, halo nevi can develop during early childhood, as early as age three.

The exact cause of halo nevi is unknown. For some reason, the body's immunologic system, the antibodies and cells involved in fighting off germs, begins destroying pigment cells in the halo nevus. Approximately 30 percent of people with halo nevi are also predisposed to vitiligo, another disorder in which the body's immune system attacks its own pigment cells (see Chapter 13).

If the central mole looks benign, no treatment is ordinarily necessary. Complete disappearance of the mole and repigmentation of the surrounding halo occurs about 50 percent of the time. But in general this process may take between eight months and eight years. If the central mole appears atypical in any way, your child's doctor may recommend a biopsy.

Benign Juvenile Melanoma

These days, just alluding to melanoma is enough to frighten all but the most stoic of parents. Although *benign juvenile melanoma* may occasionally be confused with malignant melanoma both clinically and microscopically, it is, fortunately, a perfectly benign condition. For that reason, most physicians today prefer to call it *Spitz nevus,* after the doctor who first described it.

Spitz nevi may develop in a child any time between ages three and thirteen; the vast majority appear before puberty. They are usually solitary, smooth, hairless, round or oval nodules that have a rather distinctive pink or reddish brown color and may be covered with a fine network of broken blood vessels. Typically, they vary from about ⅛ inch to ½ inch in diameter. On the arms and legs, these nevi may be mottled tan or black and possess a warty surface and irregular border, an appearance sometimes mistaken for malignant melanoma (see Chapter 13). After an initial growth phase, most Spitz nevi remain unchanged into and throughout adulthood. However, some change into ordinary, dome-shaped (intradermal) nevi. Simple surgical removal, which permits microscopic confirmation, is both diagnostic and curative.

Lentigines

Lentigines (singular: *lentigo*) are small, flat, frecklelike, circular blotches, tan, brown, or black in color. Their more even and darker coloration distinguishes them from ordinary freckles (see page 58). Ranging in size from under ⅛ to ¼ inch in diameter, lentigines may appear anywhere on the body, including the mouth and conjunctiva of the eyes. Although they first appear during childhood, they increase in number during adulthood. The color of lentigines results from the presence of more melanocytes and greater amounts of pigment in neighboring cells.

Although lentigines that appear later in life tend to persist, those that develop during childhood usually fade considerably or disappear entirely over time. Except for cosmetic reasons, these lesions require no treatment. However, because certain more serious conditions have been associated with numerous lentigines, if your child has many of them or if you've noticed that many have suddenly developed, you should consult your pediatrician.

"Misplaced" Pigment Cells

In Chapter 3, you learned that melanocytes are normally located in the basal layer of the epidermis (the uppermost layer of the skin). On occasion, they group in other skin layers, giving rise to a variety of spots and bumps.

The *blue nevus* is one such spot. Dark blue or bluish black, blue nevi get their distinctive color from the scattering of light as it passes to the deeper, abnormally situated melanocytes. They may be present at birth or develop any time thereafter. Typically, they are round or oval, smooth, and flat or dome-shaped lesions; more than one may be present in the same individual. Most blue nevi range in size from about ¼ to ½ inch in diameter. Females develop them twice as often as males.

Although blue nevi may show up anywhere on the skin, the most common sites are the buttocks, the tops of the hands and feet, and the sides of the arms. Once fully developed, they rarely change throughout life. With time, however, some may fade and flatten a bit.

By and large, blue nevi are perfectly harmless growths. Nevertheless, because of their intensely dark, bluish black coloration, they can be mistaken for malignant melanoma. In addition, there is a rare but real chance for certain types of blue nevi to become malignant. For these reasons, your pediatrician or dermatologist may suggest that your child's blue nevus be removed and examined under the microscope; happily, the cosmetic result of removal is generally quite satisfactory.

Mongolian spots are a second condition stemming from misplaced melanocytes. These deep brown, slate gray, or blue-black patches, which range in size from ¼ inch to 6 or more inches in diameter, are typically found on the buttocks, small of the back, and, less commonly, on the shoulders, flanks, back, and lower legs. As a rule, mongolian spots are *congenital*, that is, the child is born with them. Although they occur in only 10 percent of white infants, they are seen in 70 percent of Hispanics, 80 percent of Orientals, and 90 percent of blacks. Because the vast majority of mongolian spots fade as the child approaches puberty, patience is all the therapy needed.

The *nevus of Ito* and the *nevus of Ota* are two closely related conditions resulting from "misplaced" pigment cells. The nevus of Ito is a patchy, irregularly bordered, slate gray to bluish discoloration of one side of the face, most commonly the forehead, temple, and cheek. The nose and the whites of the eyes may also be involved, and, in more extensive cases, the nevus can extend into the retina and the mouth. Fifty percent of the children with this condition were born with it; the rest develop it during adolescence. The vast majority of cases are seen in Oriental females.

For all practical purposes, there are no differences between the nevus of Ito and the nevus of Ota, except that the skin staining in the nevus of Ota involves the sides of the neck, shoulder, and collarbone or wingbone (scapula). Occasionally, both nevi occur simultaneously.

Like mongolian spots, both the nevus of Ito and the nevus of Ota are entirely harmless and require no treatment. Although some degree of spontaneous fading occasionally occurs, unlike mongolian spots, these conditions do not clear completely. Many therapies, including surgery and grafting, have been tried, but no consistently effective treatment is currently available; for those who are severely troubled, satisfactory water-fast masking cosmetics (see Chapter 12) are available.

JUVENILE XANTHOGRANULOMA

Juvenile xanthogranuloma is another harmless problem of infancy and childhood whose name is far more imposing than the actual condition. The face and scalp are the typical locations for these firm, rubbery, dome-shaped growths. One or more may be present, ranging in size from pen point to about ½ inch in diameter. At first reddish and later turning orange-brown, the majority develop before the child's first birthday; on rare occasions, a child is born with them.

Sometimes a doctor may need to perform a biopsy to confirm the diagnosis of juvenile xanthogranuloma. But because these growths generally disappear spontaneously within one to two years of their development, little more attention is needed. When they develop within the eye, however, they can cause considerable damage. Prompt attention by an ophthalmologist (eye specialist) is strongly recommended.

FRECKLES

Known as *ephelides* (singular: *ephelis*) by doctors, *freckles* are typically flat, light brown or reddish spots. They are such a common skin condition that you probably have no difficulty recognizing them at a glance. I describe them here only to contrast them with the other colored, frecklelike spots described earlier.

Usually ranging from the size of a pencil point to ¼ inch in diameter, freckles are especially common during childhood, generally making their appearance somewhere between the ages of two and four. Their color is attributed to an increase in the amount of pigment dispersed through the upper layer of the epidermis, rather than to an increase in melanocytes.

The tendency to freckle runs in families and is especially pronounced in fair-skinned children with red or reddish brown hair. By and large, freckles favor heavily sun-exposed regions, such as the nose, cheeks, shoulders, and upper back. Characteristically, they fade during the winter and enlarge and darken during the summer. Because the majority of sunscreens currently available permit some degree of ultraviolet light to penetrate to the skin, they are generally inadequate for preventing freckling.

Freckles are perfectly harmless, and often disappear entirely in adulthood, so therapy is not needed. However, for older children or adults who are troubled by them, they may be lightened with cryosurgery or with strong peeling acids, for example, trichloroacetic acid (see Chapter 3). The repeated application of milder peeling agents, such as glycolic acid, may also be helpful.

CAFÉ AU LAIT SPOTS

Light brown in color, as suggested by the French phrase *café au lait* (literally, coffee with milk), these spots are found in as many as 10 to 20 percent of normal children. They may appear anywhere on the body. One or more are frequently present at birth, although far less often they can appear within the first year of life. In general, café au lait spots increase in size and number with time. *Von Recklinghausen's neurofibromatosis* (see Chapter 13), a serious multisystem disorder, must be considered whenever five or more café au lait spots larger than ½ inch in diameter are discovered.

Varying in size from about ½ inch to as much as 1 foot in diameter, café au lait spots can be thought of as giant freckles. Because the spots are harmless by themselves, therapy of any kind, except perhaps use of camouflage cosmetics, is unnecessary.

POSTINFLAMMATORY PIGMENTARY CHANGES

In general, after any episode of skin injury, irritation, allergy, or infection, the affected site becomes temporarily discolored. When the area turns darker than the surrounding skin, the condition is called *postinflammatory hyperpigmentation*. When the spot is lighter, it is referred to as *postinflammatory hypopigmentation*. Postinflammatory hyperpigmentation is by far the more common and is believed to result from increased melanin production following inflammation. Although perfectly harmless, postinflammatory hyperpigmentation may persist for several weeks to months after the causative inflammation has completely subsided. And, in general, these dark spots fade more slowly in darker-skinned children.

When fading proceeds too slowly, or when the discoloration is in a very noticeable location, such as the face, your child's doctor may recommend the use of mild antiinflammatory creams, such as Hytone, Westcort, or Locoid, to speed the healing process. Alternatively, the doctor may prescribe topical hydroquinone-containing bleaching preparations (for instance, Melanex solution or Eldopaque cream), which lighten the affected skin by blocking the production of melanin. Unfortunately, bleaching agents often take months to work, and their benefits may be completely reversed by even one episode of unprotected sun exposure. (In other words, outdoors sunscreens must be applied at all times.)

It is paradoxical that resolving inflammation sometimes leads to abnormal lightening of affected skin. Precisely why the same type of inflammation or infection leaves one child darkly blotched and another with lightish patches is not completely understood. Loss of color is believed to result from a temporary incapacity of affected skin cells to accept normal pigment granule transfers from melanocytes. The condition is otherwise harmless. And, when left alone, skin color usually returns to normal in a few weeks to a few months.

In very fair-skinned children, areas of abnormal lightening are often inconspicuous. In darker-skinned children, however, any loss of pigment can be a source of considerable embarrassment, especially when it appears on the face. In such instances, skin dyes and masking makeups of the kind recommended for use in vitiligo (see Chapter 13) may be tried until the condition abates spontaneously. In the final analysis, in either hyper- or hypopigmentation, a tincture of time (and patience) remains the best remedy.

6

OH, THOSE PESKY
DIAPER RASHES

Any parent who has ever cared for an infant with diaper rash knows what torment these pesky irritations can be—for parent and child. The rash can disturb your baby's sleep (and yours, too, naturally) and can turn even the sweetest tempered baby cranky and irritable. Diaper changes become painful and trying for parent and child. Fortunately, there are measures you can take to reduce the likelihood of the problem or its severity should it occur. Now might be a good time to review the essentials for cleansing and diapering given in Chapter 1.

Studies have indicated that as many as 16 percent of infants get diaper rash at some point, making it the most common skin eruption in infants and young children. The peak time for its development is sometime between the ages of six and twelve months. Unfortunately, this means that, despite your best efforts, there is a strong chance that your baby, at one time or another (and, if you're really unlucky, several times), will suffer from diaper rash.

Although the precise causes of diaper rash are not known, several theories have been proposed. For one thing, changes in the child's diet usually take place after the first half year, specifically, switching from breast to bottle feeding and starting solid foods.

The result is an altered composition of the urine and feces that is believed to be more irritating to the skin. After the first year, the daily frequency of urination and defecation decreases, which may account for the drop in the incidence of diaper rash at that time.

Diapering is unquestionably an efficient means for containing urine and stool. Nevertheless, the practice appears to be at odds with nature, which did not intend skin to be confined for long periods in such an inhospitable way. Within the warm, dark, tropical environment of the diaper, genetic, mechanical, chemical, allergic, and infectious factors may all come into play to contribute to diaper rashes.

By acting as physical barriers to the evaporation of moisture, diapers retain wetness and lead to overhydration of the skin. Once this occurs, the stage is set for further problems, because wet skin is much more easily irritated by friction than dry skin. In fact, it takes twice as much energy to cause frictional irritation in dry skin than in wet. Also, overly wet skin is more easily penetrated by irritating substances, such as detergents and industrial chemicals. Last, but certainly not least, wetness is conducive to the overgrowth of harmful germs.

It is not surprising that urine and fecal soilage also play their parts. Whereas normal skin tends to be slightly acidic (the so-called acid mantle), the skin within the diaper area becomes abnormally alkaline. This alkalinity, the result of bacterial breakdown of urine into ammonia, further increases skin susceptibility to penetration. Urine may also damage through the more direct skin-dissolving effects of its urea content. Finally, compounding the problem further, fecal enzymes, in prolonged contact with the skin, may also be highly irritating.

Diaper rash, or *diaper dermatitis,* as dermatologists prefer to call it, has many causes. The term is merely an umbrella category for many kinds of rashes that can appear in the diaper area. In subsequent chapters, a number of common infections and inflammations are discussed that affect many skin areas, including the diaper region. These include atopic dermatitis, seborrheic dermatitis, and psoriasis, to name just a few. This chapter, however, is confined to conditions that, either directly or indirectly, are specifically related to wearing diapers, in other words, conditions strictly meriting the label *diaper dermatitis*. By this definition, intertrigo, irritant contact dermatitis, miliaria, yeast infection, and granuloma gluteale infantum are true diaper rashes. And, although these conditions may resemble one another, their causes and treatments may vary greatly.

INTERTRIGO

Intertrigo is simply any irritation that results from a combination of wetness, heat, and sweating. Typically, the affected skin is chafed, mildly to angrily red, and occasionally oozing. The usual areas for this problem are those where skin folds overlap, such as where the thighs join the pubic region and between the buttocks. Bacterial overgrowth and contamination in these areas are not unusual.

Prevention is the best form of treatment (see Chapter 1). The use of ultra disposable diapers, frequent diaper changes, and gentle cleansing with a sensitive skin cleanser (for example, Moisturel sensitive skin cleanser) followed by a light dusting with cornstarch or talcum powder (for instance, Zeasorb) are effective measures for reducing the likelihood of intertrigo. When the condition is severe, your child's physician may prescribe a mild topical corticosteroid cream (see Chapter 7) for a few days to clear the inflammation. And, if bacterial infection should occur, the doctor may add a topical or oral antibiotic.

IRRITANT CONTACT DERMATITIS

Irritant contact dermatitis, a nonallergic form of contact dermatitis, is one of several eczemas that are discussed in greater detail in Chapter 7. Here it is enough to say that the term refers to irritation resulting from direct contact with harsh chemicals or substances. Contained by diapers, both urine and feces may become important irritants. Although infant rashes around the anus are often attributed to feces, and those in the genital region to urine, the frequent mixing of the two can make it difficult to pinpoint the greater culprit.

In general, the more frequently your infant stools in his diaper, the more likely he is to develop diaper rash. And if your baby has diarrhea, he is three to four times more likely to get diaper rash. From what has been said, the reason is clear. Feces contain certain digestive enzymes secreted by the pancreas, as well as bile salts, produced by the liver. The enzymes are especially irritating and also make your child's skin more sensitive to other substances, such as detergents and soaps.

It is interesting that breast-fed infants are generally less prone to diaper dermatitis than bottle-fed babies. This fact has been attributed not only to differences in the content of the stool but to the types and numbers of microorganisms colonizing the intestines. As a rule, the feces of breast-fed infants tend to be more acidy than those of bottle-fed infants and contain fewer urine-degrading bacteria. Levels of fecal enzymes also tend to be lower.

Irritant contact dermatitis of the diaper area can take several forms. The eruption may vary in appearance from wrinkled, parchmentlike redness to small, pimplelike bumps. Tiny blisters and erosions; large, deeply ulcerated bumps that may be as much as ½ inch in diameter; or any combination of these may also occur. The rash typically appears over areas that project outward: the buttocks, the insides of the thighs, the pubic bone, and the scrotum. In contrast to intertrigo, the skin fold areas are usually spared in irritant dermatitis. However, in severe cases, they may also be involved. Peculiar red bands often found where the diaper borders the skin are called *tidemark dermatitis*. These marks are thought to result from either repeated cycles of drying and wetting or the concentration of irritants at these areas by diaper or elastic constriction.

Preventing and treating irritant contact dermatitis involve the measures already described for simple intertrigo. To acidify the urine, some physicians recommend feeding the child cranberry juice. Before considering this, however, check with your pediatrician.

Miliaria

From Chapter 4 you may recall that *miliaria* (*heat rash* or *prickly heat*) is by no means restricted to the diaper region. However, the moisture-entrapping nature of this body area makes it especially prone to this problem. Some investigators have suggested that certain bacterial secretions in this area subject to microbial overgrowth may interfere with or block the sweating apparatus, thereby provoking the condition.

Similar to their appearance elsewhere on the body, the lesions of miliaria of the diaper area are small, individual, reddish, pimplelike bumps or pimple-blister combinations. The sites where they may occur are the same as those for irritant contact dermatitis. Itching is often intense, making the infant quite irritable.

Prevention and treatment require keeping the region cool and dry. In more severe cases, oral antihistamines, such as those mentioned for eczema (see Chapter 7), may be needed. Rarely, a mild topical corticosteroid cream (see Chapter 7) will be needed to clear the rash and control the symptoms.

Yeast Infection

Candida albicans (or *Monilia*), a microscopic yeast, is a normal inhabitant of the lower gastrointestinal system. And, as a result of its spilling out onto the skin around the anus, it also normally colonizes the diaper area. When skin contamination is unusually high, the likelihood of diaper rash increases sharply. These yeasts, believed responsible for vaginal yeast infections in adult women and a variety of other skin and nail problems, produce substances that digest skin and promote inflammation below the skin surface.

The appearance of the candida diaper rash is probably the most distinctive of all the diaper rashes. Beginning as clusters of reddish, pimplelike bumps and pustules, the lesions eventually merge into a sharply bordered, beefy red eruption. The skin folds are typically involved, a useful clue to diagnosis. The presence of isolated pustules and red bumps, known as *satellite lesions,* outside the main body of the rash is another helpful diagnostic clue. But, even when severe, the candida rash characteristically remains restricted to the diaper area. Its border is often composed of rings of white scales. Burning, itching, and tenderness are common accompaniments and make diaper changes a nightmare.

Candida dermatitis should be suspected in any case of diaper rash that does not respond to the usual conservative measures of diaper area care (see Chapter 1). It should also be suspected when diaper rash follows a course of antibiotics given for some unrelated condition. (By suppressing the normal microbial inhabitants of the gastrointestinal system, antibiotics allow the unwanted overgrowth of certain organisms, often candida.)

The diagnosis of candida diaper rash can frequently be made by observation alone. When necessary, microscopic examinations and cultures may also be performed. Contaminating bacteria often join forces with candida to aggravate the condition. When this possibility is suspected, your child's doctor may order bacterial cultures.

Once the diagnosis is established, a specific topical anticandidal antibiotic, known as nystatin cream or Mycolog, may be prescribed. More broad-spectrum antifungal creams, such as Exelderm, Mycelex, Spectazole, or Micatin, may also be used. A mild topical steroid cream, such as Hytone, Aclovate, or Westcort cream, may be added to soothe the area, reduce inflammation, and hasten healing of raw skin. Finally, when infection is resistant to therapy or when candida is also found elsewhere on the body (for example, in the mouth), a one- or two-week course of an oral anticandidal antibiotic liquid, Mycostatin suspension, may be prescribed. Naturally, all other measures previously described for diaper area care should be rigorously followed.

Granuloma Gluteale Infantum

Although *granuloma gluteale infantum* may be a separate entity, it is widely held to be a variation of a candida infection. As its name states in a Latin mouthful, this rash consists of nodules (large, high bumps). Reddish purple in color, these nodules generally range in size from $1/4$ inch to more than 2 inches in diameter. The lower buttocks are the most common location; however, the groin, lower abdomen, penis, and even areas outside the diaper region, such as the armpits and neck, are sometimes involved. To the untrained eye, this condition can be alarming in appearance, and, by the more experienced eye, it is sometimes confused with certain malignancies. Happily, the condition is entirely benign.

A biopsy is occasionally needed to confirm the diagnosis of granuloma gluteale. Left untreated, lesions usually clear slowly over several months. Injections of steroids directly into each area (intralesional injections) can hasten clearing, although this measure is seldom required. When candida is shown to be present, antifungal agents should be added to the treatment regimen.

7

ALL KINDS OF ECZEMAS

Eczema, an imposing-sounding word, is often used interchangeably with *dermatitis,* which literally means "inflammation of the skin" (*derma* = skin; *itis* = inflammation). Usually named for their presumed causes, eczemas are generally intensely itchy, reddish skin rashes. Several significant types are common to children. However, if your child is diagnosed as having an eczema, you needn't panic. Many treatments are now available for managing eczemas, and some types can even be prevented altogether simply by eliminating known triggering factors.

Before I describe specific eczema conditions, a definition of inflammation is in order. *Inflammation* is a complicated and dynamic process in which the body's natural defenses attempt to handle attack by allergens, irritants, or germs. Natural defenses include a host of chemicals, hormonelike substances, antibodies, and special cells. The results of this struggle are responsible for the telltale signs of inflammation, which include redness, heat, pain, and the diminished ability of affected areas to function normally. Contrary to a popular notion, inflammation does not automatically imply infection. Infections (see Chapter 10) are only one type of inflammatory process. Eczemas are another.

ATOPIC ECZEMA

By far the commonest of all childhood skin conditions, *atopic eczema* affects approximately 3 percent of children. Dermatologists describe it as an "itch that rashes," meaning that the skin may at first appear perfectly normal, despite intense itching. Soon, however, frenetic scratching and rubbing provoke the rash, which further intensifies itching and sets up the so-called itch, scratch, itch cycle. This process is the reverse of most other eczema rashes, in which the rash precedes the itch. (Note: By itself, the word *atopy* refers to a personal or family history of asthma, hay fever, or eczema, and it is estimated that between 30 and 50 percent of children with atopic eczema eventually develop either asthma or hay fever.)

Atopic eczema is divided into three stages: infantile, childhood, and adult. The first stage usually begins when the infant is between two and six months of age. Areas of intense itching, redness, tiny blisters, oozing, and crusting typically appear first on the cheeks, forehead, and scalp and later extend symmetrically down the chest and back and onto the arms and legs. By the time children are age two or three, half the cases of infantile eczema disappear on their own.

In the remaining cases, the condition progresses to the childhood stage, when the oozing and crusting are replaced by drier, darker, scalier, and thicker patches (a process known as *lichenification*). At the same time, the sites typically shift to the inner folds of the arms and knees and to the wrists and ankles.

Pleats and creases are two other conditions commonly found in childhood atopic eczema. *Pleats* are extra lines or grooves that develop below the lower eyelids. Also called *Morgan's folds* or *Dennie's pleats,* they are most commonly present at birth and are believed to result from the accumulation of small amounts of inflammatory fluid in the soft tissues under the eyes. Abnormal skin *creases* consist of fine, deepened, normal skin markings and additional fine lines on the palms. They are believed to result from abnormal dryness and thickening of the skin. Although they tend to persist throughout life, both pleats and creases are harmless.

Half of those who suffer from atopic eczema in childhood will experience complete clearing sometime before the onset of puberty; the remainder will go on to the adult stage, which usually consists of red or reddish brown bumps, dry patches, and skin thickening. This stage can persist well into the individual's twenties or even throughout life. The hands, feet, face, neck, and folds of the arms and legs become the most frequent trouble spots.

A variety of factors are known to aggravate (not cause) any stage of atopic eczema. Physical stresses, such as dramatic shifts in temperature and humidity, and fevers, colds, flu, and allergy attacks have all been known to trigger flare-ups in predisposed children. Nervous tension is also a well-recognized factor.

Because soap and water can be very drying, particularly to sensitive, atopic skin, you should bathe your child less frequently and limit the amount of time spent in the bath. Tepid water is preferable to hot water. Select sensitive skin cleansers (for instance, Moisturel sensitive skin cleanser and Lowila Cake) rather than harsher toilet soaps or antibacterial soaps (see Chapter 1). In general, avoid dressing your child in scratchy, woolen materials; stick with soft cotton clothing. Swimming in chlorine pools, which are especially drying, should be restricted whenever the eczema is active. Finally, because extremes of temperature and humidity can be aggravating, air-conditioning in the summer and humidification in the winter months can be beneficial.

Naturally, if your child suffers from atopic eczema, he should be under the care of a dermatologist or pediatrician experienced in dealing with the problem. In general, the main goals of any treatment plan are to reduce the occurrence of flare-ups, minimize dryness and itching, and prevent bacterial contamination of sore or broken skin.

One of the most frequent questions I am asked is whether diet plays any role in atopic eczema. Although specific foods do not appear to cause the condition, certain ones have been known to provoke attacks, especially in infants and small children. (In adults the link is much weaker.) Potential troublemakers include cow's milk, eggs, fish, wheat products, nuts, and citrus fruits. Under the guidance of your child's physician, a trial period of avoiding suspected offending foods may prove worthwhile.

Another frequent question is whether airborne allergies play any role. Occasionally, dust and dust-gathering objects—pillows, carpets, and drapes, for example—are linked to worsening of atopic eczema. To minimize this possibility, you can remove carpets and drapes from your child's room and use plastic covers on pillows and mattresses. Skin testing for airborne allergens and desensitization shots, however, are rarely of any value. In fact, allergy shots may worsen the atopic rash.

When conservative measures fail, topical corticosteroids become the mainstays of treatment for atopic eczema. *Corticosteroids* are hormonelike antiinflammation drugs that rapidly relieve itching and clear the rash. They range in strength from mild to superpotent. Available in creams, lotions, ointments, gels, and sprays, these products are deceptive, appearing to be ordinary cold creams, moisturizers, or Vaseline-like salves. They are, in fact, potent drugs, whose prolonged or improper use can cause permanent damage to your child's skin, including abnormal thinning, mottled pigmentation, broken blood vessels, and stretch marks.

In general, creams deliver the active steroid ingredient in an aesthetically pleasing, vanishing formulation. For deeper penetration, or when more skin lubrication is desired, ointments are usually prescribed, although they are messier. For hairy areas, lotions and gels are generally best, because they penetrate to the skin surface without matting the hair.

For fear of producing unwanted side effects, many pediatricians prefer to prescribe only the least potent topical steroid formulations. But unfortunately in many cases, atopic eczema, especially when severe, does not respond adequately to such therapy. Most dermatologists would agree that a short course of high-potency topical steroids can bring about immediate symptomatic relief without producing any of the feared side effects, which generally occur after several weeks of daily use.

Once your child's skin is clear, maintenance therapy to prevent flare-ups may be recommended. This usually means switching to daily use of low-potency steroids or the occasional application of high-potency steroids, say on weekends only. This regimen is known as *intermittent, topical, high-dose pulse corticosteroid therapy*. In between steroid applications, I usually prescribe Lac-Hydrin lotion twice daily to protect and lubricate the skin.

In a very difficult-to-manage case, your child's doctor may prescribe antihistamines, such as Benadryl or Atarax, for both itch reduction and sedation. When the skin has broken down from relentless scratching or become heavily colonized or infected with bacteria, oral antibiotics, such as erythromycin or dicloxacillin, may be prescribed, after appropriate bacterial cultures of the skin have been taken. Staphylococci or streptococci are the usual culprits (see Chapter 9). When all else fails, a short course of oral corticosteroids, such as prednisone or dexamethasone (in pill or elixir form) can generally bring the condition rapidly under control.

For more information about atopic eczema, you may contact the executive director of the Eczema Association for Science and Education by writing to 1221 SW Yamhill, Suite 303, Portland, OR 97205.

Several conditions are found so frequently in children predisposed to atopic eczema that they are often considered linked to it. These include keratosis pilaris, pityriasis alba, and icthyosis vulgaris. Others, such as xerosis (excessive dryness), creases of the palms, and pleats have already been discussed.

Keratosis Pilaris

Keratosis pilaris is a very common childhood condition in which numerous tiny, spiny, reddish, whitish, or flesh-colored bumps develop on the outer arms and outer thighs. The eruption may develop by itself or frequently in association with atopic eczema or ichthyosis vulgaris (see page 75). Occasionally, the entire torso can be affected and, rarely, even the face. The appearance of keratosis pilaris has been likened to that of plucked chicken skin or gooseflesh. Protruding pores (follicles), overstuffed with keratin protein, account for the graterlike feel of the skin.

Keratosis pilaris is a harmless disease, which by itself causes no symptoms. In many children it disappears spontaneously around puberty. In some, however, it may persist well through the teens and even into the twenties and thirties. When treatment is desired, Lac-Hydrin lotion, a prescription-only moisturizing drug, can be particularly effective for softening and loosening the abnormal protein plugs. Occasionally, a mild topical steroid may be prescribed to diminish redness and inflammation.

Lichen spinulosus may be thought of as a highly localized form of keratosis pilaris. The affected area, generally only one site on the trunk or extremities, appears as a round, oval, or line-shaped patch of numerous tiny, spiny bumps. Like keratosis pilaris, this condition is most commonly found in children with atopic eczema, is entirely harmless, and requires no therapy except for aesthetic reasons. It may be treated in much the same fashion as keratosis pilaris. In addition, salicylic acid–containing gels, such as Keralyt, can be helpful for thinning and softening the patches.

Pityriasis Alba

In *pityriasis alba,* numerous abnormally lightened patches of skin develop on the child's face, neck, back, upper chest, and upper arms and legs. In infants, the condition can be even more widespread. Lesions vary in size from ½ inch to several inches in diameter, and the borders of each are hazy and usually covered with a fine, powdery scale.

The cause of pityriasis alba remains unknown. However, it is believed to be some form of dermatitis (possibly atopic eczema). The depigmentation is thought to result from an interference with the normal processes of pigment transfer and tanning within the epidermis in response to sunlight. For this reason, the condition is often first diagnosed after a period of sun exposure. As a rule, pityriasis alba responds rapidly to topical corticosteroid therapy. But, although the depigmentation is reversible, it can take from weeks to months to return to normal.

Ichthyosis Vulgaris

Ichthyosis vulgaris is by far the mildest and most common of a group of inherited scaling disorders. It has been estimated that somewhere between 1 in every 250 and 1 in every 1,000 infants is born with this tendency. It is passed from one generation to the next and can show up anytime after the age of three months. The term *ichthyosis* is derived from the Latin prefix *ichthy*, meaning "fish," and in this condition platelike, fishlike scales are found on the outsides of the arms and especially on the legs. The bends of the arms and the backs of the knees are characteristically spared. In more extensive cases, small, white, branlike scales may cover the cheeks, forehead, and upper areas of the body. It is not uncommon for children with ichthyosis also to have keratosis pilaris and accentuated creases on the palms of their hands. Cold and chapping weather and low humidity indoors can be especially rough on ichthyotic skin.

Treatment is basically directed at keeping the skin well lubricated. Here again, the high-potency, prescription-only moisturizing lotion Lac-Hydrin, has proven especially useful. For milder cases, a lower-concentration, over-the-counter product, such as Lac-Hydrin 5 lotion, may be used. For children sensitive or allergic to lactic acid preparations, urea-containing emollients, such as Aquacare-HP or Carmol 10 lotion, can be tried. Cold-air humidifiers or several flat pans of water placed near radiators can be important during the wintertime. For more information on this and other ichthyotic disorders, you may contact the Foundation for Ichthyosis and Related Skin Types, Inc. (FIRST), P.O. Box 20921, Raleigh, NC 27619-0921.

SEBORRHEIC DERMATITIS

Seborrheic dermatitis, totally unrelated to atopic dermatitis, is another common inflammatory condition found in infants. The name comes from the fact that the eruption occurs in the *sebaceous areas,* those parts of the body having the greatest concentrations of sebaceous glands: the scalp, face, area behind the ears, breastbone, armpit, and groin. The name, however, is misleading because there is no evidence that the condition is related to diseased oil glands or to glandular overproduction.

A hereditary tendency appears to exist for seborrheic dermatitis, whose precise cause remains unknown. In the infant, hormones passed from the mother while the infant is still in the womb are thought to play a significant role. A yeastlike organism that normally inhabits the skin, *Pityrosporum ovale,* may be another triggering factor.

In infants, seborrheic dermatitis usually begins on the scalp, some time between the second and twelfth weeks of life. This is frequently referred to as cradle cap (see Chapter 4). In more widespread cases, the rash may progress downward to involve the forehead, ears, eyebrows, nose, chest, back, and groin. Sometimes a dry scaliness, rather than oiliness, is found. The condition is very unusual during later childhood, although it frequently recurs after puberty.

Infantile seborrheic dermatitis, which seldom itches, ordinarily clears by itself in a few weeks or months. When treatment is needed, over-the-counter antidandruff sulfur- and salicylic acid–containing shampoos, such as Sebulex, used two or three times a week, or chloroxine lotion (Capitrol), also used two or three times a week, effectively control most cases. Tar shampoos, such as T/Gel or Ionil T, are also effective. Warmed mineral oil massaged gently into your baby's scalp and then rinsed out, or Baker's P&S liquid left in place overnight before rinsing can help dislodge tightly adherent scales and crusts. And a soft brush or just your fingertips (nails trimmed, of course) are fine for combing them out.

For the most resistant cases, a short course of a topical corticosteroid lotion for the scalp and cream for the body may be prescribed. Once seborrheic dermatitis is brought under control, maintenance therapy, similar to the kinds advised for atopic eczema, may be suggested.

CONTACT DERMATITIS

As the name suggests, *contact dermatitis* is an inflammation of the skin resulting from contact with some offending substance, known as a *contactant*. When the rash is provoked by a highly irritating substance, dermatologists call it *irritant contact dermatitis*. Chemicals known to trigger this reaction include those found in harsh soaps, detergents, bleaches, solvents (such as turpentine and carbon tetrachloride), acids, alkalis, bubble bath products, urine, stool, foods, and even saliva. Factors such as how long the skin was in contact with the chemical and whether the skin was healthy at the outset or wet at the time of contact (wetness or perspiration usually worsen the problem) determine the severity of the reaction. It is not uncommon to find a family predisposition to contact dermatitis.

When a rash results from an allergic response to a contactant, it is known as *allergic contact dermatitis*. Poison ivy dermatitis is probably one of the best-known examples of this type. Other common contact allergens include nickel (in jewelry), neomycin (in triple antibiotic ointments), formaldehyde (in wash-and-wear and permanent-press clothing), ethylenediamine (a stabilizer), and parabens (preservatives). Foods are also well-known causes of contact allergy around the mouth.

Development of a contact allergy necessitates both repeated exposure to an offending substance and a mature immune system. Thus, children younger than three, with their still developing immune systems and, generally, little experience of repeated exposures, seldom develop allergic contact dermatitis. This does not hold true, however, for children between the ages of three and eight.

Your child's doctor can usually diagnose either type of contact dermatitis on the basis of the appearance and distribution of the rash and of the history of contact exposure to known potential allergens or environmental irritants. In the earliest stage of the reaction, affected areas are swollen, deeply red, and covered by tiny, often oozing blisters. Later, crusting, scaling, and thickening of the skin occur, and blistering becomes less pronounced. If contact with the offending substance continues, marked thickening, cracking, and scaling may completely replace blistering.

Typically, irritant dermatitis begins *immediately after* exposure to the culprit chemical. By contrast, the first episode of allergic contact dermatitis generally occurs within a week to ten days following exposure and as early as eight to twelve hours after each subsequent exposure. Although typically just one exposure to a harsh substance is enough to trigger irritant contact dermatitis, many prior (sensitizing) exposures are needed to trigger allergic contact rashes. Nevertheless, for both irritant and allergic contact dermatitis, avoiding the suspected troublemaker is the best therapy.

Poison Ivy Dermatitis

Poison ivy dermatitis (also called *rhus dermatitis*) is by far the most common allergic contact dermatitis in the United States. The term *poison* is entirely misleading. More precisely, the culprit, an oily resin that coats the plant's leaves, twigs, stems, and roots, is an allergen. It is so potent that an estimated 70 percent of people exposed to it eventually develop the allergy.

Poison ivy is found throughout the United States. Poison sumac, found in woody and swampy areas east of the Mississippi, and poison oak, found on the West Coast, are relatives of poison ivy capable of causing the same allergic rash. A linelike group of small blisters, appearing where the plant has brushed against the skin, is typical of these rashes, and its presence often points your child's doctor to the diagnosis.

Obviously, the best way of dealing with these plant allergens is to avoid contact. The Boy Scout manual's advice—"Leaflets three, let them be"—remains a sound rule to follow. Susceptible children should, if possible, be kept away from areas known to harbor poison ivy, and all children should wear protective clothing at all times in high-risk areas. For particularly allergic children, I suggest the use of Ivy Shield (made by Interpro, Inc.). This lotion, which you apply before going outdoors, is used by the Forestry Service and has proved helpful in preventing or minimizing the reaction. Another lotion, Wonder Glove (formerly Dermofilm, made by Global Consumer Services, Inc.), may also be helpful for reducing the effects of contact in susceptible children.

Once exposure has occurred, the best therapy is to wash off the resin immediately. Do not wait more than ten minutes. Although soap and water are okay, isopropyl rubbing alcohol is far better for dissolving the resin. Because the resin may retain its allergic potential from months to years, everything worn at the time of exposure, including sneakers, should be laundered.

Cool compresses followed by the application of calamine lotion make the best first aid in mild cases. Over-the-counter antiitch products containing benzocaine or diphenhydramine should be avoided, because these chemicals may themselves be allergenic in a lot of children. In more severe cases, your child's doctor may prescribe topical steroids. Sprays, gels, and creams are preferable for their drying effects in the acute early phases. Occasionally oral steroids, usually prednisone or dexamethasone, are prescribed. Although the eruption generally clears quickly with oral steroids, the dose usually must be tapered over a two- to three-week period to prevent rebound flare-ups that can be as severe as the original condition.

Shoe Dermatitis

Shoe dermatitis is another very common form of allergic contact dermatitis in children. The numerous chemicals used in the manufacture of shoes include plasticizers, tanning agents, adhesives, cements, and dyes, many of which are potential allergens. Approximately three-quarters of all cases of contact shoe allergy, however, have been linked to the following agents: dichromates, mercaptobenzothiazole, tetramethylthiuram, and monobenzyl ether of hydroquinone.

Shoe dermatitis typically starts over the tops of the big toes and eventually develops over the surfaces of the other toes. Involved areas become red and thickened and, in severe cases, turn wet and crusted. Shoe allergies are much less common on the heels and soles because of their thicker, more resistant skin. In particularly sensitive children, however, the entire bottoms of their feet may also be affected. It is not uncommon for shoe dermatitis to be mistaken for severe athlete's foot fungus infections (see Chapter 10). Examining the web spaces between the toes can be helpful to distinguish the two. Fungal infections characteristically attack the web spaces, whereas contact allergy does not.

The severity of the rash determines the kind of therapy. In mild cases, a low-potency topical corticosteroid will probably be sufficient. In more severe instances, soaking in aluminum acetate (Burow's solution or Domeboro packets) or tannic acid solutions (2 tea bags in a quart of water), coupled with the use of high-potency topical steroids, may be needed. If secondary bacterial infection is present, antibiotics are required.

Naturally, as with poison ivy, prevention is the best form of management for shoe dermatitis. Children with shoe allergies would do better to avoid wearing leather shoes as much as possible and wear fabric sandals or slippers instead. Open sandals are preferable in warm weather and indoors, and canvas-topped sneakers, vinyl tennis shoes, all-vinyl shoes, unlined moccasins, and Celstic (nonrubber) box toes make suitable shoe substitutes. If inner soles prove to be the problem, have your shoemaker replace them with cork insoles, Johnson's Odor-Eaters, or Dr. Scholl's air foam pads, using plain Elmer's Glue in place of rubber cement.

Perspiring feet not only directly irritate shoe dermatitis but are also responsible for leaching chemicals from shoes. Therefore, you must make every effort to keep your child's feet dry. Socks should be changed frequently. Dusting shoes and socks with Zeasorb powder to reduce wetness and provide a barrier to allergens may also help. In severe cases, your doctor may prescribe aluminum chloride drying agents, such as Xerac AC, Drysol, and Hi-Dri. These products are believed to work by temporarily clogging the sweat pores. For maximal effectiveness, they are best applied at bedtime to work overnight.

Once an acute episode has cleared, your child's dermatologist may recommend *patch testing* to determine the precise chemical or chemicals responsible for the shoe allergy. In this test, a series of Band-Aid-type patches containing suspected allergens is applied to a nonhairy area of skin, generally the back or the forearm, and left in place for forty-eight hours. Screening trays containing common shoe and rubber contact allergens are available for this purpose. The patches are then removed to see which chemicals have reproduced the eczema condition. When circumstances warrant, the physician may also cut out pieces of material from your child's shoe or sneaker, moisten them with water, and patch them directly to the skin. Either way, patch testing necessitates no breaks in the skin or injections, making it quite acceptable to children.

ODDBALL ECZEMAS

Dishidrotic Dermatitis (Dishidrosis)

As though the name *dishidrotic dermatitis* or *dishidrosis* were not weighty enough, this condition sometimes goes by the unwieldy designation *pompholyx*. Basically, it is an eczema that affects only the hands and feet. The cause of the condition is still unknown, although it is more common in children with a personal or family background of atopic diseases (asthma, hay fever, or eczema). It frequently occurs in high-strung children.

Redness and crops of tiny, straw-colored, fluid-filled vesicles erupt symmetrically on the soles of the feet, palms of the hands, and sides of the fingers, accompanied by burning and itching. Although these tiny blisters occasionally merge, more often they gradually dry up, leaving fine scaling in their wake. Attacks of dishidrosis generally clear spontaneously within a few weeks but may recur as frequently as several times a year; these episodes are often linked to periods of heightened emotional stress.

The word *dishidrotic* implies some form of malfunctioning of the eccrine sweat glands (see Chapter 3); however, no such abnormalities have been conclusively established in this condition. Nonetheless, excessive sweatiness of the palms and soles often accompanies the eruption.

In mild cases, drying medications, such as those used in shoe dermatitis, may be helpful. Daily soaks in tar solutions, such as

Balnetar (2 capfuls in a basin of water once or twice daily for fifteen minutes), may be helpful for reducing inflammation and alleviating itch. More often, topical corticosteroid creams are prescribed to suppress the eruption.

Once this eruption has been cleared, you should encourage your child to follow a few simple measures to reduce the frequency and severity of recurrences. Wearing gloves to prevent chapping is a must during the winter. And all year round, the hands should be gently washed with sensitive skin cleansers, such as those recommended in Chapter 1. Routinely apply a hypoallergenic moisturizer several times daily, especially after hand washing. For tough cases, the prescription-only moisturizing drug Lac-Hydrin lotion, applied twice daily, can be particularly effective. For children sensitive to lactic acid, 10 to 20 percent urea creams or lotions may be tried (Aquacare, Carmol). Finally, Wonder Glove (formerly Dermofilm) makes a good skin protectant, especially when applied before your child swims in a chlorinated pool or has anticipated contact with nontoxic paints, ceramics, clay, or glues.

NUMMULAR ECZEMA

Nummular eczema, whose name is derived from the Latin *nummulus*, meaning "a coin," appears as coin-shaped plaques. Starting as small pimply or blistery bumps, the eruption enlarges to form sharply bordered, round or oval patches, usually on the outsides of the arms, hands, legs, and feet. In more advanced cases, it can involve the chest, back, and buttocks, rarely even the face. Individual spots may vary from ½ inch to several inches in diameter. Although a link between nummular and atopic eczema has been speculated, no connection has ever been firmly established.

Itching and general skin dryness commonly accompany an outbreak. It is not surprisingly that cold and dry environments can aggravate the rash or even provoke it in susceptible children.

Excessive washing or bathing, harsh cleansers, and scratchy woolen clothing also tend to aggravate the problem.

Treatment consists of protecting your child from these aggravating factors and minimizing dryness by the use of gentle cleansers and moisturizers, as described for dishidrotic dermatitis (see page 82). For severe outbreaks, a short course of a high-potency topical steroid cream rapidly clears most cases. For maintenance (after clearing), I prefer intermittent, topical, high-dose pulse corticosteroid therapy, as described in Chapter 7, especially during the drying winter months.

Lichen Striatus

Lichen striatus is another common but odd childhood eczema, in that it typically affects just one arm, or one side of the neck, chest, back, or buttocks. Individual spots are tiny, flat-topped bumps that are pink or flesh-colored and covered by a very fine, silvery scaliness. In dark-skinned or black children, these bumps may appear underpigmented. Individual lesions may be pinpoint-sized, although they often merge to form linelike plaques several inches in diameter. The linear distribution is often a tip-off for the doctor.

Lichen striatus is rarely found in infants, making its first appearance in children somewhere between the ages of three and ten years. Girls are affected two to three times as often as boys. Attacks come on suddenly, reach a maximum severity in a few days to several weeks, then disappear on their own within six to twelve months. Because this condition causes no symptoms, no treatment other than reassurance is necessary. However, if your child is old enough to be concerned about his or her appearance, your physician may prescribe a topical steroid to speed clearing.

Frictional Lichenoid Dermatitis

Frictional lichenoid dermatitis is still another odd eczema, in which the rash occurs only on the elbows, knees, and backs of the hands. It affects boys, mostly between the ages of four and twelve. Consisting of a dense grouping of flesh-colored or pinkish, flat-topped bumps, it develops during the spring and summer months, primarily in boys with a personal or family history of atopy. Because of its seasonal incidence, your doctor may refer to this condition as *summertime pityriasis* (scaling).

The eruption, which seldom itches, usually clears by itself in several weeks, only to recur the following spring. Because it appears at a time when children play outdoors, and because many cases have been associated with playing in sandboxes, this eczema has been called *sandbox dermatitis*. Leaning on the elbows and knees is believed to be the cause.

Prevention and maintenance measures for frictional lichenoid dermatitis are simple; they consist of protective clothing to reduce frictional irritation and the use of high-potency lactic acid or urea compounds, like Lac-Hydrin and Carmol-10. Although seldom required, topical steroids may also be prescribed to hasten clearing.

8

PSORIASIS AND OTHER INFLAMMATIONS

Eczemas, especially atopic eczema and poison ivy dermatitis, are the most common skin problems in children, but they are by no means the only kinds of skin inflammations that can occur. The list includes psoriasis and a host of less frequently heard of disorders; however, only the more common ones are discussed in this chapter. In the not too distant past, disorders such as psoriasis were difficult to clear up and often quite disabling. Today, parents and their children both are spared much of the distress in coping with these problems, for, although total cure still eludes us in many instances, medical advances have made these inflammations far easier to treat and far less daunting to live with.

PSORIASIS VULGARIS

Psoriasis is an extremely common, noncontagious disorder affecting an estimated 3 percent of all Americans. At present, this translates into roughly 8 million people, with approximately

150,000 new cases diagnosed each year; over one-third develop this disorder during childhood or adolescence, and of those a significant number show the first signs and symptoms before the age of five. Among children, the number of girls affected is twice that of boys. Don't be put off by the designation *vulgaris,* which is not intended to be pejorative. The word simply means "common" or "garden variety." A number of other forms of psoriasis exist, some of which are touched on in the following pages.

Many researchers believe there is a hereditary predisposition to psoriasis. A child having one parent with this condition is three times more likely to develop it than one with no family history of it. Studies in twins also support this notion. If one twin develops psoriasis, the other is usually more than 70 percent at risk.

The fundamental abnormality of this condition is the tremendous increase in the rate at which epidermal cells are produced and shed. Ordinarily, this process takes about twenty-eight days; in psoriasis, it takes only three or four, resulting in the thickened, heavily scaled patches characteristic of the disease.

Surmounted by thick, whitish, micalike scales, lesions of psoriasis are typically round, reddish patches with sharp borders. When removed, these scales, which are the hallmark of the condition, leave behind many pinpoint bleeding spots. This is called *Auspitz's sign* and is highly suggestive of psoriasis to your child's doctor. You should not, however, intentionally remove the scales.

Psoriatic patches, which can range in size from the width of a droplet of water to many inches in diameter, may develop anywhere on the body, including the nails and scalp. Although only one area may be affected, it is more usual for many spots to be symmetrically distributed over the body. The most characteristic locations are the regions over the bony pressure points of the knees, elbows, shins, and lower back, as well as the scalp. In extreme cases, the entire body may be affected at once.

Attacks often begin in areas that have been scratched, cut,

burned, sunburned, or inflamed by other conditions, such as atopic eczema or seborrheic dermatitis (see Chapter 7). This is known as the *Koebner phenomenon*. Infections, particularly strep throat, and the ingestion of certain medications, such as beta blockers (for example, propanolol) and indomethacin, may also trigger flare-ups.

Psoriasis has a number of variants. One, known as *guttate psoriasis*, generally occurs in children. More than two-thirds of the time, it follows by one to three weeks some form of upper respiratory infection. *Guttate* means "droplike," and the lesions in this condition may measure from no larger than the point of a pen to as much as $\frac{1}{8}$ inch in diameter. These lesions are usually symmetrically located over the chest, back, thighs, and upper arms. Another variant, referred to as *seborrhiasis* or *sebopsoriasis,* may appear in the same locations seborrheic dermatitis (see Chapter 7) is typically found. Occasionally, even your child's doctor may have difficulty distinguishing the two. In general, ordinary seborrheic dermatitis is confined within the hairline and responds fairly quickly to treatment. By contrast, psoriasis spills onto the forehead, temples, and nape of the neck and is quite resistant to therapy. When the armpits, the groin, and the creases around the genitals and buttocks are involved, the condition is known as *inverse psoriasis.*

Still another type of psoriasis involves the nails. Studies indicate that *psoriatic nail dystrophy* (psoriasis of the nails) occurs in somewhere between one-quarter and one-half of all sufferers. Pitting, or the development of pen-point-sized depressions in the nail, is the most common manifestation. Crumbling, grooving, discoloration, separation of the nail from the bed below, and the accumulation of thick, whitish debris under the nail are more extreme manifestations of this condition.

Psoriasis also has pustular variants. In one mild type, pustules from $\frac{1}{8}$ to $\frac{1}{4}$ inch in diameter develop on the hands and feet only. A much more serious type, known as *generalized pustular psoriasis of von Zumbusch,* a condition that may affect both infants and small children, is a suddenly occurring, potentially fatal, widespread pustular eruption accompanied by high fever. In this form, sheets of red, pustule-studded skin replace previously normal skin, particularly in the bends of the arms and legs, in the finger webs, around the fingernails, and in the genital region. Even the mouth and tongue can be involved.

Your child's doctor will usually be able to diagnose ordinary psoriasis or its variants on the basis of the history and the appearance and distribution of the rash. When the diagnosis is not so clear, a biopsy may be recommended for confirmation.

Psoriasis is a chronic disorder, for which there is no cure at present. Typically, it has ups and downs—referred to as *spontaneous remissions* and *recurrences.* For this reason, the doctor must tailor treatment to the type and severity of your child's problem. It is thus advisable to place your child under the care of a dermatologist experienced in the management of psoriasis and its complications. She or he can maintain a constant liaison with your child's pediatrician, so that optimal total care can be delivered.

Topical steroids (see Chapter 7) are generally the first line of therapy for most types of psoriasis. Superpotent steroids, such as Ultravate and Temovate, or high-potency topicals, such as Maxivate or Diprosone, used for courses of from one to two weeks, can be extremely helpful in bringing about clearing in many cases, with few side effects. Once clearing is achieved, intermittent, topical, high-dose pulse corticosteriod therapy, as outlined in Chapter 7, can be initiated for maintenance.

Resistant patches of psoriasis can be treated with occlusive dressings, that is topical steroids covered with a plastic wrap (for instance, Saran Wrap) dressing to lock moisture in and increase penetration of the medication. A commercially available steroid-impregnated tape, Cordran Tape, may instead be prescribed. More recently, an occlusive dressing, Actiderm (Squibb), was approved for use in treating plaques of psoriasis either alone or in combination with a topical steroid. Although resolution generally occurs quite slowly when plain occlusion is used, prompt clearing can be achieved by the injection of a small amount of a steroid directly into the base of the plaque.

Tar preparations, possessing both antiitch and antiinflammatory properties, have long been employed in the treatment of psoriasis. Messy to use and staining to clothing, they fell into relative disuse when the more effective and aesthetically pleasing topical steroids came along. These days, however, more agreeable tar-based products are available. For soaking in a bath, two capfuls of Balnetar may be used, and, for daily direct application, Estar gel may be recommended in place of topical steroids. With tars, clearing tends to be slow, usually taking several weeks.

Anthralins, another class of nonspecific antiinflammatory and antiitch medications, have also been around for decades. Like tars, they fell into disfavor because of their messiness and staining of clothing and skin. In answer to those problems, Drithocreme was recently introduced and its efficacy demonstrated. For convenience, your child's dermatologist may suggest SCAT therapy, whose name stands for *s*hort-*c*ontact *a*nthralin *t*herapy. This consists of only one twenty-minute application each day. However, a fair amount of patience is required, because clearing takes time.

Ultraviolet light has also proven beneficial in treating psoriasis. Although sunburn should be avoided, gradual exposure to the sun during the spring, summer, and early autumn can be helpful in bringing about and maintaining remissions. Alternatively, ultraviolet light from artificial sources in combination with the application of tar-based medications (Goeckerman regimen) or anthralin formulations (Ingram method) may be prescribed. Both methods employ ultraviolet B radiation, and, depending on the severity of the condition, your child can receive treatments at a hospital as either an inpatient or outpatient, at a clinic, or at the doctor's office. With a doctor's prescription, home ultraviolet light units are available for purchase through National Biological Corporation (Twinsburg, OH), the Daavlin Company (Bryan, OH), and the Cooper-Hewitt Corporation (Erlanger, KY). In most cases, these regimens require several weeks to bring about clearing.

PUVA, or *p*soralens, high-intensity, *u*ltraviolet *A* light therapy, involves the prior administration of oral or topical ultraviolet light–sensitizing chemicals, known as psoralens, followed by exposure to selective, highly concentrated UVA radiation. Treatment takes place once or twice a week until clearing is achieved; then a maintenance schedule tailored to the individual child is begun. PUVA therapy is rarely advised for pre-teens. Of course, with any ultraviolet light therapy, including natural sun tanning, the short-term benefits must be weighed against the long-term risks of ultraviolet exposure (see Chapter 2). You should discuss this trade-off openly with your child's physician.

A number of other psoriasis therapies merit brief mention, although the details are beyond the scope of this chapter. These include the use of potent systemic medications, such as the folic acid antagonist methotrexate; the vitamin A derivative and relative of the strong antiacne drug Accutane, Tegison (etretinate); and, most recently, the potent immunosuppressive agent cyclosporine A. The decision to use any of these drugs is serious. Fortunately, because of the effectiveness of the treatments mentioned earlier, the use of any of these therapies in young children is rarely necessary.

For more information on psoriasis, you may contact the National Psoriasis Foundation at P.O. Box 9009, Portland, OR 97207.

LICHEN PLANUS

Like psoriasis, *lichen planus* is an inflammatory condition whose precise cause remains unknown. Although this is largely a disease of adults, a fairly substantial percentage of cases occur in infants and young children.

Ranging from pinpoint size to ½ inch in diameter, the small, shiny, flat-topped, reddish or purplish papules of lichen planus are fairly distinctive. The base of each papule may take the form of a square, rectangle, or other polygon, but the top is typically perfectly flat. Groups of lesions may merge to form large plaques. The wrists and ankles are favored locations, and the mucous membranes, particularly the mouth, are involved in 70 percent of cases. The Koebner phenomenon described on pages 88–89 may also occur in lichen planus. Severe itching is common.

There are more than half a dozen variations of lichen planus. Ringlike, linelike, wartlike, and even blistering types can occur. At times, the disorder can also attack the nails and scalp, leading to considerable tissue destruction, permanent scarring, and irreversible nail distortion or nail and hair loss.

In most cases, your child's doctor will be able to diagnose lichen planus solely on the basis of the history and appearance of the lesions. A biopsy is rarely needed. Because most cases clear within eight to sixteen months, some within a few weeks, reducing itching is the primary focus of treatment in children. In most cases, a short course of high-potency topical steroids will help clear the lesions and reduce the itch. Antihistamines, such as hydroxycine (Atarax) or diphenhydramine (Benylin), may be added when necessary for their antiitch and sedating properties. Despite treatment, the skin of previously affected sites may remain abnormally darkened for weeks to months (postinflammatory hyperpigmentation, see Chapter 5). Between 10 and 20 percent of children with lichen planus suffer at least one recurrence.

URTICARIA (HIVES, WHEALS)

Hives, or wheals, as they are also known, are tiny, fluid-swollen bumps that can occur singly or in groups just about anywhere on the skin or mucous membranes. Ranging in size from as small as a pencil eraser to the width of a dinner plate, they may look absolutely frightening, especially when they involve the soft, elastic tissues around the eyes, lips, and genitals. Although usually causing itching, stinging, or burning, hives occasionally produce no symptoms or signs besides swelling. Although new hives may continue to appear for days to weeks, individual hives last no longer than twenty-four hours.

An estimated 20 percent of people will develop a hive attack sometime in their lives, and such episodes are designated acute or chronic, based on how long new hives continue to appear. By definition, *acute* attacks last under three weeks, whereas *chronic* attacks exceed six weeks. A hormonelike chemical, *histamine,* produced in special cells in the skin known as mast cells, is believed to be largely responsible for hiving. Release of this hormone can be precipitated directly by chemicals in certain foods or drugs, or indirectly by exposure to substances to which a child is allergic.

Foods and infections are the two most common causes of acute urticaria. Nuts, egg whites, berries, tomatoes, citrus fruits, fish, pork, and seasonings such as catsup, mustard, and mayonnaise are among the food culprits most frequently associated with episodes of hives, which can begin from minutes to hours after ingestion. Upper respiratory infections, chicken pox, and rheumatic fever, and drugs, such as aspirin, penicillin, sulfa, and codeine, may also trigger acute hive attacks. So can insect bites (see Chapter 10). Few of us have been lucky enough to escape the nasty stings of mosquitoes, blackflies, hornets, wasps, bees, and yellow jackets. Each sting site is actually a hive.

Foods, infections, drugs, and bugs must also be considered in cases of chronic urticaria. In addition, superficial fungal and yeast infections (see Chapter 9), bladder and kidney infections, tooth abscesses, and chronic sinusitis have all been known to provoke persistent hive attacks in susceptible individuals. But still other causes must be explored. For example, in atopic children (see Chapter 7), there is frequently a familial predisposition to hives (mold allergy being the most common trigger). An under- or overactive thyroid may also be a cause.

Mechanical factors may likewise contribute. In *cholinergic urticaria*, for example, tiny hives surrounded by a white or reddish halo appear within sixty to ninety minutes after sweating, sun exposure, hot baths, or blushing. In another condition, known as *cold urticaria*, hives are triggered by cold or if the body becomes chilled. Yet another type, *pressure urticaria*, can be provoked by simple pressure, such as that produced by a tight elastic waistband. And in *dermatographia* (sometimes called *skin writing*), a condition that affects about 7 percent of all people at some point in their lives, welts appear after ordinary rubbing or scratching. Finally, even ultraviolet light can elicit hives in some children, a disorder known as *solar urticaria*.

The best treatment for any form of hives is elimination or avoidance of the cause. However, given the enormous number of environmental triggering agents, it sometimes takes a Sherlock Holmes to discover the culprit. Your child's doctor will start by taking a detailed history, including questions about diet and medications taken for other conditions. It is important that you mention even such seemingly innocuous substances as vitamin supplements, because the fillers, preservatives, and dyes in these products have been known to cause hives. If airborne or seasonal allergens are suspected, the doctor may order special blood and urine tests, and occasionally X rays and scratch tests. (Testing for food allergens, other than by trial and error, is unreliable and in most cases unproductive.)

Unfortunately, in perhaps as many as 90 percent of children with chronic hives, no specific cause can be identified, and outbreaks are labeled *idiopathic urticaria*, a fancy name for "hives of unknown cause." In these instances, treatment consists of general attempts to reduce emotional stress and exposure to heat or tight clothing, and the use of antihistamines to control the symptoms. Atarax, Chlor-Trimeton, and Benadryl are three of the more common antihistamines that have proven safe and effective for children. Periactin is the drug of choice for cholinergic urticaria.

Although antihistamines help relieve itching and swelling, they are also sedating. Thus, while they can be especially helpful at bedtime, they can make your child groggy and cranky during the day. Because they generally take about ninety minutes to begin to work, antihistamines are best used prophylactically on a daily basis to prevent attacks rather than once an attack has started. How long preventive therapy must be maintained is variable and must be tailored to the individual child. Recently, two nonsedating antihistamines, Seldane and Hismanal, were approved by the FDA. It is hoped that their value and safety for children will stand the test of time.

In more severe cases of hives, especially those involving swelling in the throat and around the windpipe, emergency care is critical, and injections of epinephrine (adrenaline) can be lifesaving. Oral steroids may also be needed.

DRUG ERUPTIONS (DERMATITIS MEDICAMENTOSA)

Given the enormous numbers of drugs that are currently available, it is hardly surprising that many cause adverse reactions in the skin. *Drug eruptions* (technically, *dermatitis medicamentosa*), which tend to cover much of the body, may take several forms. Commonly, they are measleslike in appearance. But, they may take the form of flat, reddish rashes, reddish bumps, hives, erythema multiforme (see page 98), or lichen planus (see page 92), among others. Although almost any drug is capable of causing a drug eruption, some are more likely to do so than others: penicillin and penicillin derivatives (ampicillin, amoxicillin, and dicloxacillin), cephalosporins (Keflex, Velosef, and Duricef), and barbiturates.

In general, diagnosis of a drug eruption is likely whenever an itchy, widespread rash follows within hours to days after exposure to a drug. When the diagnosis is less clear, a biopsy may be recommended for confirmation. For mild cases, withdrawing the offending drug is the best form of treatment and usually leads to complete clearing in about a week. For more fully developed drug eruptions, topical antiitch lotions and steroids may be prescribed, along with some form of antihistamine, such as Atarax. Systemic steroids are reserved for more severe cases.

Fixed Drug Eruption

Fixed drug eruption is a quirky kind of drug allergy, in that one, or at most only a few, round or oval patches develop in the same location or locations on the skin or mucous membranes each time the offending drug is taken. The reason for the body's odd reaction is not known. Lesions are usually brownish or dusky brownish purple and occasionally blister. Common allergens known to cause fixed drug eruptions include penicillin, salicylates, antihistamines, barbiturates, ipecac, and Dilantin. Subsequent reexposures to the offending drug frequently incite reactions more severe than the original episode.

Although a biopsy is sometimes needed to establish the diagnosis, the history of the allergy and a physical examination of the child are ordinarily enough to suggest it strongly. Except for avoiding the culprit drug, no therapy is generally needed. In their wake, fixed drug eruptions leave brownish discolorations (postinflammatory hyperpigmentation, see Chapter 5) that may take many weeks to fade.

Erythema Multiforme

Erythema multiforme is an umbrella term for another group of pre-sumed allergic disorders whose most severe variants are particularly common during childhood. Appearing frequently in the spring or autumn, the typical eruption favors the palms and backs of the hands, the soles and heels of the feet, and the outer arms and legs; the skin, and mucous membranes may also be affected. As with hives (see page 94), foods, drugs, underlying malignancies, and certain infections have all been known to trigger the condition. Cold sores (fever blisters) are probably the single most common trigger of erythema multiforme and usually precede its onset by two weeks. It is interesting that many of the drugs that provoke hives can precipitate erythema multiforme.

The hallmark of erythema multiforme is the so-called *iris* or *target* lesion, which is a reddish, bull's-eyelike ring. Lesions may also be flat, dull red, dusky, hivelike, pimplelike, and even blistering, hence the designation *multiforme*. In mild cases, the eruption is the only manifestation. In more severe cases, low-grade fevers, muscle aches, and generalized tiredness are common. In *Stevens-Johnson syndrome,* the most severe and potentially life-threatening variant of erythema multiforme, high fever and denuded or completely open blisters often necessitate hospitalization for supportive care; the eye, mouth, and anogenital regions are frequently involved.

The diagnosis of erythema multiforme is usually confirmed by biopsy. Treatment depends on the severity of the eruption. As with hives, finding the causative agents and avoiding further contact with them are of paramount importance. Depending on the circumstances, antihistamines and oral or intravenous steroids may be needed. For temporary numbing, painful oral sores may be treated with diphenhydramine elixir (Benylin) and viscous Xylocaine 2% (Lidocaine) swished around the mouth and spit out several times daily.

SCHÖNLEIN-HENOCH PURPURA

Sometimes called *anaphylactoid purpura*, this is another allergic type of disorder that mainly affects children between three and ten years of age. The medical term *purpura* simply means bruises or black-and-blue marks, areas where bleeding has taken place within the skin. As a rule, ordinary bruises from a fall or a bang are perfectly smooth. By contrast, those in this disorder are bumpy. Known as *palpable purpura*, these bruises are an important clue to an allergic blood vessel inflammation. In this condition, which often follows an upper respiratory infection, intense inflammatory damage to blood vessels is responsible for the leakage of fluid and blood corpuscles into the surrounding tissues.

In typical cases, crops of bruised-looking flat spots, bumps or welts, and occasionally small ulcerations develop over the buttocks and outsides of the arms and legs, especially over the knees and elbows. Alarming swelling can sometimes occur on the scalp, face, genitals, hands, and feet. As new crops of bruises appear, older ones fade, leaving brownish discolorations. In general, the older the child the less severe the attack.

Unfortunately, body systems besides the skin may also be involved. Kidney inflammation occurs in about half the children affected, and gastrointestinal problems, liver irritation, and arthritis may also develop.

A biopsy is usually needed to confirm the diagnosis of Schönlein-Henoch purpura. Blood and urine tests are also frequently ordered to assess damage to other organs. Bed rest and a short course of oral corticosteroids are sometimes recommended to control the acute symptoms. The majority of children with this condition recover fully without further complications.

MUCHA-HABERMAN DISEASE

There's no getting around this mouthful, because its other name is even worse: *pityriasis lichenoides et varioliformis acuta* (PLEVA). Mucha-Haberman disease, which largely affects children and young adults, also involves inflammation around blood vessel walls, leading to leakage of blood and fluid. Allergy to medications or infection are the speculated causes.

The eruption typically appears in waves of symmetrically distributed round or oval, reddish or brownish, flat or bumpy lesions, ranging from pinpoint size to ⅛ inch in diameter. These spots soon turn into tiny blisters, which eventually ulcerate and crust over. Although the eruption can involve any part of the body, the trunk, thighs, and upper arms are the favored locations. New spots may continue to appear for several weeks to months before the condition finally clears on its own. Unfortunately, it is not uncommon for attacks to recur, generally about three years after the first episode.

A biopsy is often needed to distinguish PLEVA from a variety of other common conditions that can mimic it, such as impetigo and chicken pox (see Chapter 9), or scabies (see Chapter 10). Because its precise cause remains unknown, treatment of PLEVA is primarily directed to relieving the symptoms. Aspirin, erythromycin, topical steroids, tar, ultraviolet light, and lubrication have all been tried with varying success.

9

IF IT'S NOT ONE GERM, IT'S ANOTHER

It's a fact of life. Your child lives in a hostile world of germs. And no matter how hard you try to protect him or how attentive you are to his hygiene, it's impossible to prevent your child from putting things in his mouth, or getting kissed by adults with colds, or catching things from other children.

Were it not for the near miraculous capabilities of the body's immune system—the antibodies and special cells exquisitely designed to fight off invading germs—all of us would succumb to infection in no time. The tragic, untimely deaths of those rare children born with severe deficiencies of the immune system, or those suffering from AIDS, attest to just how effective this system is for the rest of us. And this struggle to fend off the world of germs goes on practically every minute of every day. Occasionally, however, certain germs put up a good fight and take hold, and they are the subject of this chapter.

BACTERIAL INFECTIONS

Our skin is a wonderful barrier to infection. But when it is broken by cuts, scratches, or insect bites, an avenue for bacterial infection is opened. At this point, the immune system whips into action to fight off the invaders. If it wins, no infection. If it fails, infection takes root.

Pyodermas

Impetigo contagiosa, one of several bacterial conditions known as *pyodermas* (*pyo* means "pus" and *derma* "skin"), is probably the most common superficial skin infection seen in children. As its full name suggests, it is a highly contagious condition, caused by either staphylococci or streptococci, and is referred to as a "superficial" infection because it is confined within the skin and does not penetrate into internal organs. Although it can occur anywhere on the body, impetigo usually appears on exposed surfaces, namely the face, hands, neck, arms, and legs—sites where injury is more likely to occur. The phrase *secondary impetiginization* specifically refers to impetigo that sets in after the skin has been compromised by some prior inflammation, such as eczema (see Chapter 7) or infection (for example, herpes, see page 106).

In its most typical form, impetigo begins with $\frac{1}{8}$- to $\frac{1}{4}$-inch reddish spots that quickly change into tiny, thin-walled blisters surrounded by a red border. The blisters soon rupture, discharging a clear, yellow, highly infectious fluid that dries into soft, thick, honey-colored crusts. Characteristic of impetigo, these crusts teem with bacteria eager to contaminate fingers, towels, clothing, and other children. Dislodging a crust exposes a smooth, red, weeping base that rapidly crusts again. Itching is a common symptom.

If impetigo is left untreated, satellite infections may form around the initial site, and there may be significant spread to other areas; the problem can persist for weeks. The most dreaded complication, however, is an allergic reaction that certain strains of strep organisms may trigger in the kidneys, known as *acute glomerulonephritis.* Fortunately, this complication is rare.

The diagnosis of impetigo can usually be made by the naked eye, although bacterial cultures are frequently taken to confirm the diagnosis and pinpoint the causative germ. As a rule, impetigo responds rapidly to oral antibiotics, such as erythromycin or dicloxacillin. In addition, infected areas should be cleansed with hydrogen peroxide and covered with a topical antibiotic ointment, such as Polysporin. More recently, the potent topical antibiotic ointment mupirocin (Bactroban) was approved by the FDA, and preliminary evidence suggests that it may be as effective as oral erythromycin for treating impetigo. Certainly in children it makes an effective, convenient alternative to systemic therapy.

Ecthyma is a more severe variant of impetigo in which the sores are deeper and ulcerating. Strep organisms are the usual culprits. Beginning much like ordinary impetigo, ecthyma burrows into the skin, causing considerable pain and leaving punched out or saucer-shaped scars. Treatment, which should be instituted early to minimize disfigurement, is the same as for impetigo.

Folliculitis

Infection occurring high within the shafts of hair follicles is known as *superficial folliculitis.* This condition is caused by staph organisms and primarily affects the child's scalp, face, buttocks, arms, and legs. Typical lesions, which resemble acne blemishes, are dome-shaped pustules surrounded by reddish halos and pierced in their centers by hairs. Outbreaks are usually painless and tend to appear in crops. Some children complain of itching.

Diagnosis and treatment are much the same as for impetigo, although oral antibiotics are seldom necessary. They are generally reserved for more persistent cases. Gentle cleansing with soap and water, followed by the application of a topical antibiotic lotion, such as T-Stat lotion (erythromycin), is usually sufficient for clearing inflammation and preventing further outbreaks.

Furuncles (boils) are deeply situated, painful abscesses surrounding hair follicles. More common in older children, this condition in most cases develops from a preceding episode of folliculitis. The scalp, neck, face, armpits, chest, thighs, buttocks, and genitals are favored locations. Characteristically red, tender, and boggy nodules, boils may range from ½ inch to 3 inches in diameter. Left untreated, they may burst spontaneously, leaving a contagious, blood-tinged, pussy fluid. *Carbuncles* are large abscesses that form when two or more adjacent boils merge.

Treatment for boils and carbuncles consists of frequent use of warm, moist compresses and oral and topical antibiotics. *Incision and drainage* (surgically opening and draining boils under local anesthesia) is the treatment of choice once they soften and come to a head ("point"). Pain relief is immediate after drainage.

Cellulitis

Generally starting a day or two following some type of injury or break in the skin, *cellulitis* is a common bacterial infection of childhood that affects the deeper, fatty tissue of the skin. Staphylococci and streptococci are the usual causes in older children, whereas *Hemophilus influenzae* (*H. flu*, for short) is more common in children younger then two. Infected areas are angry red, warm, swollen, and tender; however, in *H. flu* cellulitis they tend to be dusky red or purplish red. Children with cellulitis generally run high fevers and are quite sick. Blood poisoning (or, more correctly, bacterial contamination of the bloodstream from infected sites) is a serious complication and must be treated aggressively as soon as possible.

The diagnosis of *H. flu* cellulitis can usually be made on clinical grounds. If necessary, bacterial culture confirmation can be obtained by *needle aspiration* (withdrawing infected tissue fluids through a needle inserted to the level of the infection). Injection of antibiotics, most often dicloxacillin, amoxicillin, cephalexin, or erythromycin, is the treatment of choice. The response to treatment is dramatic; clinical improvement occurs within twenty-four to seventy-two hours.

Erysipelas is a form of cellulitis that occurs most frequently in infants and very young children. The infection is located higher up within the skin than ordinary cellulitis. Following a break in the skin, a patch of redness begins, then enlarges to become a painful, hot, tender, shiny, bright red plaque. The border of the plaque is typically very sharp. The scalp and face—especially the cheeks and the bridge of the nose—are favored sites of attack, although erysipelas can appear anywhere on the body. Infected children often run high fevers and are quite ill. Streptococci are by far the most common cause of erysipelas, making oral penicillin the drug of choice for treatment. Severe cases may require hospitalization and intravenous antibiotic therapy.

Scarlet Fever (Scarlatina)

Largely affecting children between one and ten years of age, *scarlet fever* is a throat infection, usually a strep throat, that is accompanied by both a body rash (called an *exanthem*) and a mouth rash *(enanthem)*. The rash is produced by a toxin secreted by the bacteria. Occasionally, certain staphylococcal skin infections may give rise to a scarlet fever–like eruption known as *scarlatina*. Fall, winter, and early spring are the prime seasons for this condition.

After a one- to seven-day incubation period, scarlet fever begins abruptly with sore throat, fever, headache, exhaustion, and vomiting. About the same time, the mucous membranes of the mouth turn a bright red. Shortly thereafter, the tongue usually becomes swollen and coated and begins to resemble a ripe strawberry. This condition has been aptly nicknamed *strawberry tongue.* Flat reddish and purplish spots also begin appearing on the soft palate, the fleshy mucous membrane at the rear of the roof of the mouth.

Within forty-eight hours, a pinpointlike, sandpapery, reddish rash develops on the trunk and later spreads over the entire body. For some reason, the eruption *(circumoral pallor)* characteristically spares the area around the mouth. At the same time, because of fragile capillaries and leakage of blood and fluids, horizontal darkened lines *(Pastia's lines)* appear in the bends of the arms. After about five days, the rash is replaced by widespread, branlike scaling—a hallmark of scarlet fever. Complications are uncommon but include serious allergic conditions affecting the heart and kidneys *(rheumatic fever* and *poststreptococcal glomerulonephritis,* respectively).

A presumed diagnosis of scarlet fever can be confirmed with throat cultures and special antibody tests for streptococci. Penicillin is the drug of choice, and prompt treatment is required to prevent or minimize complications. Dicloxacillin is the preferred drug for staphylococcal scarlatina.

VIRAL INFECTIONS

Herpes Simplex

Herpes simplex is one of the most common infections in human beings. Two closely related types of herpes viruses have been identified: *HSV I* and *HSV II.* In the past, it was believed that HSV I only infected sites above the waist and HSV II below the waist. Today, we know that either type may cause infection anywhere on the body. In general, infections are acquired from close contact with family members or friends carrying the virus and are transmitted through touching, kissing, and even sharing towels and eating utensils.

Primary herpes of the mouth and oral cavity, or *herpetic gin-givostomatitis,* is the most common herpes virus infection in children, peaking in incidence sometime between one and five years of age. Active infection generally begins about three to five days after a child has been exposed to an infected individual or carrier. At this time, the mouth and oral tissues become covered with fragile, viral blisters, which soon break. The lips, palate, and gums may all be involved. In as many as 15 percent of affected children, eating and drinking become extremely painful. Although the majority of sufferers have no other symptoms, fever, swollen lymph nodes, and generalized aches and pains may accompany the outbreak.

Unfortunately, although research continues, no cure yet exists for herpes infections. Primary infections usually clear by themselves in two to three weeks. In the interim, symptoms can be alleviated with analgesics, such as acetaminophen (Tylenol), oral rinses with diphenhydramine (Benylin elixir), and topical anesthetics, such as Chloroseptic spray. If necessary, your child's doctor may prescribe the topical anesthetic viscous Xylocaine 2%. Drinking liquids must be encouraged to prevent dehydration.

Neonatal herpes occurs when infants are born to mothers with active genital herpes infections close to or directly involving the birth canal. Death, serious neurologic complications, and mental retardation are among the potential tragic consequences of this infection. Although there is only an estimated 50 percent chance of transmitting the virus to the infant as it passes through a herpes-infected vagina, a cesarean section is usually performed to avoid this risk.

Recurrent Herpes Simplex Virus Infections

Herpes infections unfortunately remain for life. When the acute condition subsides, the herpes virus goes into hiding in the nerves near the spinal column closest to the site of infection. It may stay inactive for weeks to decades before reappearing. In this phase, the infection is said to be *latent*.

Reactivation, a process in which the virus resurfaces to the skin, can be triggered by a variety of factors. These include unprotected sun exposure, nervous tension, injury, illness, and fever. *Cold sores* or *fever blisters* are actually recurrent herpes simplex viral infections of the lips. The frequency of recurrences is variable; some people may have only one episode the rest of their lives; others may have them nonstop. In most cases, the frequency of attacks decreases after age thirty-five.

Unlike the blisters in primary herpes, those in recurrent infections tend to be smaller and arranged in a group on a tender, reddish base. After only one to three days, they become pussy and later crust over. In all, they last only seven to ten days. Tingling, itching, burning, and other odd sensations may be felt in the affected area anywhere from three to seventy-two hours before the blisters appear, and nearby lymph glands may become swollen. But, in general, there are no other accompanying symptoms. Recurrent attacks typically appear at or near the site of previous outbreaks.

Diagnosing recurrent herpes infections is usually not difficult. For confirmation, your child's doctor may take a viral culture or perform a special microscopic analysis of a skin scraping from a blister, known as a *Tzanck smear*. Biopsies are seldom required.

Treatment is directed to shortening the course of the infection and reducing discomfort. Cleaning affected areas with hydrogen peroxide, followed by applying a topical antibiotic (for instance, Polysporin or Bacitracin ointment) will help prevent bacterial contamination. A five-day course of acylovir (Zovirax) suspension may be prescribed to reduce viral shedding and speed healing. For children who are plagued by frequent recurrences, Zovirax may also be advised for preventive daily use. To date, no vaccine is available to prevent primary attacks or abort recurrences, although research continues in these directions.

Afflicting 20 percent of the population at large, *canker sores,* or *aphthous stomatitis,* are one of the most common inflammations of the mouth. Although viruses are not believed to play any causative role in this condition, it is mentioned here because canker sores are often confused with the lesions of recurrent herpes virus infections. The condition is not contagious, and genetic, allergic, and nutritional factors have all been postulated as causes.

In contrast to herpes infections, which generally involve the gums, roof of the mouth, and outsides of the lips and nostrils, canker sores involve the inside linings of the lips and cheeks. Ordinary canker sores begin as small, oval or round, reddish swellings. Within a day, these rupture, leaving thin, white or yellow, membranelike coverings surrounded by reddish halos. Canker sores range from 1/8 inch to 1 1/4 inches in diameter. Attacks generally last from ten to fourteen days. Recurrences, which may be either infrequent or continuous, are typical. As with herpes, sufferers may experience a prior tingling or pain in the area of the mouth where the sores will soon erupt.

To reduce the likelihood of canker sore recurrences or to limit aggravating an ongoing problem, avoid giving your child abrasive or spicy foods, such as potato chips, catsup, and mustard. And brushing teeth must also be gentle. For relief of symptoms, over-the-counter antihistamine rinses, such as Benylin, and topical anesthetic sprays, such as Chloroseptic, can be helpful. More troublesome cases may require prescription anesthetics, such as viscous Xylocaine 2%, and rinsing with tetracycline elixir. Occasionally a short course of a high-potency topical steroid ointment (for example, Maxivate) may be added to reduce inflammation further.

Warts (Verrucae)

Warts (technically *verrucae*) are benign skin growths caused by *human papilloma virus (HPV)* infection of the epidermis. So far more than fifty subtypes of HPV have been identified, some possessing the potential for malignancy. Being viral, warts are contagious. And because injury promotes inoculation of the virus, warts typically develop in areas subject to the greatest trauma—the hands, arms, and feet, where there are often breaks in the skin.

Warts are generally named for either their actual physical appearance or their site of attack. For example, ordinary, rough-surfaced, and thickened warts are designated *verrucae vulgaris,* and smaller, smoother ones are classed as *flat warts (verrucae plana).* Those infecting the heels and soles of the feet are known as *plantar warts (plantar* meaning "foot," and having nothing whatever to do with plant*ers* or planting); in the genital area, they are called *genital warts* (or *condylomas*), and around the fingernails, *periungual (peri =* around; *unguis =* nail) warts.

Common warts can appear anywhere on the body, although most often they develop on the backs of the hands and around the fingernails. They may be yellowish tan, grayish black, or brown and typically have rough, abrasive-looking surfaces. One variant, known as *digitate* or *filiform warts,* has fingerlike or threadlike projections that make it easily identifiable. A child may develop only one wart or hundreds.

Flat warts arise primarily on the face, neck, arms, and legs. They are roundish, flesh-colored or slightly tan or brown bumps measuring between $\frac{1}{8}$ and $\frac{1}{4}$ inch in diameter. Again, one or hundreds may be present. Plantar warts are found on the weight-bearing regions of the toes, heels, and soles of the feet. Instead of growing outward, like other warts, plantar warts are pushed inward by the pressure of walking and running. As a result, they tend to be deep and painful.

By contrast with other types, genital warts are typically brownish, fleshy, cauliflowerlike growths. Warts in the genital and anal areas can also spread from warts elsewhere on the child's body and do not necessarily indicate sexual abuse.

In most cases, diagnosing warts presents little problem to the dermatologist. Confusion sometimes arises when warts become scratched, injured, or rubbed, and on the feet they may be mistaken for corns or calluses. Dermatologists search for tiny, black dots within the affected tissue (which represent wart blood vessels) and for the absence of normal skin markings. (Warts typically obliterate normal skin markings, whereas corns and calluses do not.) Rarely, a biopsy may be needed to establish the diagnosis.

Although some doctors recommend leaving warts alone in the hope that they will clear spontaneously, I have too often seen warts spread and become numerous to agree. The choice of treatment depends on the age and personality of the child, as well as the number, size, and location of the warts. The simplest treatments involve home use of combinations of mild acids, such as salicylic acid and lactic acid (for instance, Occlusal and Duofilm). Treatment often takes many weeks and is not always successful. Treatments by a doctor include the application of strong caustics, such as 50% trichloroacetic acid (or podophyllin for condylomas), cryosurgery, laser surgery, and curettage and electrosurgery. Of all, I find curettage and electrosurgery, the last option, to be the simplest and most highly effective method. Unfortunately, even under the best of circumstances, warts recur as much as 10 to 15 percent of the time.

Suggestion therapy is sometimes successful in those small children who still believe in the curative power of "magic kisses." It consists of the hocus-pocus application of smoking or brightly colored liquids, or injections of saline right into the wart. The power of the mind to enhance the body's immune system is believed to be at the root of this approach's success, as well as of the reputed cures for warts attributed to a wide range of folk remedies of the past.

Molluscum Contagiosum (Water Warts)

Molluscum contagiosum is another very common childhood skin infection caused by one of the largest-sized viruses known to infect humans. Although occasionally found in infants, molluscum is more often seen in children after the age of three. As its full name clearly states, it is contagious not only to other areas of your child's skin but to other children and adults as well. The incubation period varies from two to twenty-six weeks.

Mollusca are typically flesh-colored or pinkish, waxy-looking bumps with a central depression that makes them look something like tiny volcanoes. Ranging in size from pinpoint to an inch or more in diameter, they can infect the face (including the lips and mucous membranes), chest, back, and upper extremities, especially the folds of the arms and the armpits. One or many may be present.

Molluscum infection is fairly easily diagnosed, and biopsy is rarely needed for confirmation. Left untreated, an episode usually clears on its own somewhere between a few months and several years after appearance. Nevertheless, because it is impossible to say in which child the condition will linger or spread, I usually recommend some form of treatment. Cryosurgery and the application of 50% trichloroacetic acid are generally effective methods of destroying the warts. In the older, more cooperative child, however, the simplest techinque is to scrape them off after numbing directly with a skin refrigerant, such as Fluro-Ethyl spray.

CHILDHOOD EXANTHEMS

Chicken Pox (Varicella)

Chicken pox (or *varicella*) is a highly contagious childhood disease, with outbreaks usually coming in winter or early spring epidemics. More than 50 percent of cases occur before the age of five.

Following an incubation period of approximately ten to twenty-one days, successive crops of tiny blisters typically appear over a three- to five-day period. Because each blister sits on a reddish base and has a tiny depression in its center, the blisters have been likened to teardrops. Erosions throughout the mouth are also common. Headache, fever, and tiredness frequently accompany the rash.

In otherwise healthy children, chicken pox is generally a mild illness, and treatment is directed at reducing the fever, discomfort, and itch. Viscous Xylocaine 2% (Lidocaine) may be needed when oral discomfort is severe or interferes with eating. Your child's dermatologist may recommend calamine lotion or prescribe a compound lotion consisting of varying concentrations of menthol and phenol in a moisturizer to alleviate the itch. Oral diphenhydramine (Benylin) or chlorpheniramine (Chlor-Trimeton) may also be needed. Because of the well-known association of aspirin ingestion, childhood chicken pox, and Reye's syndrome, a severe liver ailment, aspirin should *not* be given for aches, pains, or fever; acetaminophen (for instance, Tylenol) is preferable.

Measles (Rubeola)

Despite the availability of an effective vaccine, *measles* (or *rubeola*), which was on the decline nationwide, unfortunately is once again being seen in increasing numbers. From an all-time low of approximately 1,500 cases in 1989 the number has since shot to an alarming 16,000 plus. Measles is spread from one person to another by airborne droplets.

The outbreak of the measles rash is preceded by a ten- to fourteen-day incubation period, toward the end of which come fever, chills, headaches, eye irritations, runny nose, and dry, hacking cough. *Koplik's spots,* tiny, blue-white bumps that resemble grains of salt sprinkled on a reddish background, are seen on the insides of the cheeks near the first molars. The rash begins near the hairline as reddish or purplish red spots or bumps and spreads downward to encompass the face and the remainder of the body. Large patches of rash form where spots merge. Clearing generally occurs in three to four days. Although uncommon, complications of measles include pneumonia, ear infection, severe neurologic involvement, and even death.

Diagnosing measles usually presents little problem. Treatment is symptomatic and consists of bed rest and acetaminophen (Tylenol). For prevention, live virus vaccination administered to children at fifteen months of age and again when they enter school has proven 95 percent effective. After exposure, however, gamma globulin (immune globulin) injections may prove useful to any nonimmunized child, especially when given within seventy-two hours of contact.

Rubella (German Measles)

German measles (or *rubella*) is another common childhood condition. Like ordinary measles, it is spread by airborne droplets via the respiratory tract, and it has a two- to three-week incubation period. The rubella rash, which consists of rose-pink, measleslike spots and bumps, begins on the scalp and hairline and proceeds to the trunk. Affected areas typically fade as new ones appear. German measles spreads more quickly than ordinary measles, and in children the outbreak of the rash coincides with the onset of other symptoms, including mild fever for about a day, mild sore throat, a cough, minor eye irritations, and swollen lymph glands in the neck and behind the ears.

For the vast majority of children, rubella is an innocuous condition. (But for pregnant women in the first trimester, it is an entirely different matter, highly likely to cause intrauterine infection and serious fetal complications.) The diagnosis, which is usually straightforward, may be confirmed by blood antibody tests. Treatment is directed at alleviating any symptoms. Live virus vaccination after the age of fifteen months is highly effective.

Roseola Infantum (Exanthema Subitum)

Roseola infantum (or *exanthema subitum*) is a condition of suspected (though as yet unproven) viral causation that affects children mostly between three and twelve years years of age. After an approximately one- to two-week incubation period, a sunburnlike, or slapped cheek–like rash suddenly appears on the cheeks. It is followed within twenty-four hours by a measleslike rash on the outside of the arms and legs, and, less commonly, on the chest, back, and buttocks. The eruption fades a few days later, leaving a lacy rash that may persist for days to weeks. There are rarely any accompanying symptoms. Diagnosis hinges on the typical pattern of the rash. Treatment of any kind, other than reassurance for the parents, is rarely needed.

Hand-Foot-and-Mouth Disease

The name *hand-foot-and-mouth disease* gives away a lot of information about this infection which can affect children of all ages and is caused by the Coxsackie A16 virus. (*Coxsackie* is the name of the town in upstate New York where the condition was first described nearly forty years ago.) Following a three- to six-day incubation period, the eruption begins in the mouth as small, red spots that later turn into canker sore–like blisters of varying sizes. Shortly thereafter, small, reddish, measleslike spots appear on the tops of the hands and feet, and occasionally on the palms and soles. In turn, these quickly become roundish or football-shaped blisters, each surrounded by a red halo. Fever is the most consistent accompaniment to the rash, but a flulike feeling is also common. In the vast majority of instances, the symptoms and signs disappear within a few days. Treatment is largely reassurance and acetaminophen (such as Tylenol) for the fever and flulike aches and pains.

FUNGAL INFECTIONS

Fungi are a group of microscopic plant organisms. Unlike ordinary plants, fungi lack flowers, leaves, and chlorophyll. As a result, they are unable to make their own food and must depend on decaying matter or living tissue for nourishment. Fungal infections limited to the skin and mucous membranes are known as *superficial* fungal infections.

Candidiasis (Moniliasis)

Candida or *monilia,* as it is also frequently called, is a yeastlike fungus that normally colonizes the mouth, gastrointestinal system, and vagina. Under ordinary circumstances, it is prevented from causing problems by our immune defenses. However, when the delicate balance between our immune system and these organisms is upset, for example, after oral antibiotics or corticosteroids have been taken for other reasons, candida may begin attacking the host tissue. By and large, the warm, moist folds of the groin, buttocks, and thighs are the favored sites of attack.

Candida may also infect the mouth. In this condition, known as *thrush,* grayish white, curdlike clumps of fungal material adhere tightly to the tongue, palate, inner cheeks, and gums. Beneath the curds, the mucous membranes are intensely red and inflamed. When candida infects the moist corners of the mouth, the problem is known as *perleche* (or *angular cheilitis*).

Your doctor can confirm candida infection by examining skin scrapings under a microscope and taking a culture from the affected area. The gentle removal of the curds with a Q-tip and an application of nystatin (Mycostatin suspension), an anticandida antibiotic, will usually clear up the problem. If not, or if the problem recurs frequently, oral ingestion of Mycostatin may be necessary. It is important not to stop treatment as soon as the area looks and feels better. Ideally, treatment should be continued until repeat fungal cultures indicate that the organism has been entirely eradicated. Repeated applications of zinc oxide ointment coupled with ketoconazole (Nizoral) cream will usually clear perleche in a few weeks.

Newborns are unusually susceptible, and candida skin infections in infants may be present at birth, as a result of contamination in the womb, or appear within several days of birth, as a result of passage through a contaminated birth canal. Such infants may also become oral or intestinal carriers of the yeast, in whom the mouth and intestines become sources for future saliva or stool contamination of the skin and mucous membranes.

In some newborns, candidal lesions may involve the head, face, neck, chest, back, arms, and legs, typically sparing the diaper region. In others, infection may begin in the area around the anus and go on to involve the buttocks, groin, and then more distant sites. In either case, the eruption starts as reddish spots that eventually turn to pustules before drying up and clearing over a few weeks in most cases. A diagnosis of suspected newborn candidiasis can be confirmed by the microscopic and culture methods mentioned above. Broad-spectrum antifungal agents, such as Exelderm cream, or more specific agents such as Nizoral cream, are effective in clearing these conditions. For more resistant or persistent cases, oral Mycostatin suspension may be needed.

Tineas

Tineas, a second major grouping of superficial fungal infections, are caused by a variety of distinct fungi. As a rule, the site of involvement determines the name of the condition. For example, a fungus infection of the feet is called *tinea pedis* (*pedis* means "foot"); a fungus infectin of the entire body is referred to as *tinea corporis* (*corporis* meaning "body"), and so on.

Commonly known as *ringworm, tinea corporis* is an infection of the nonhairy areas of the body, such as the face, chest, back, arms, and legs. Fairly symmetrically located, the spots tend to be oval-shaped, scaly patches with a clear center and a sharp, scaly, blistery, or pustular border. The ringlike shape explains the familiar name of this condition, but the infection has nothing to do with worms of any kind. It is not uncommon for tinea corporis to take the form of a widespread, scaling rash rather than the ring form.

Tinea Pedis (Athlete's Foot)

Tinea pedis (or *athlete's foot*) is estimated to affect as many as 90 percent of the U.S. population at some point in their lives. Despite its popular name, however, the condition probably has far more to do with sweaty sneakers, sweat-retaining rubber, or synthetic (acrylic and polyester) socks than with any particular sport or athletics.

Athlete's foot may take three forms. In one form, it is restricted to the area between the fourth and fifth toes, where it causes scaling and cracking. In a second form, it leads to blistering on the soles of the feet. And in a third type, it causes scaling and/or redness in the so-called *moccasin distribution,* on the heels, soles, and around the sides of the feet.

In many instances, diagnosis of athlete's foot requires skin scrapings for microscopic and culture studies to distinguish it from severe dry skin, psoriasis, eczema, or allergic dermatitis. Broad-spectrum antifungals, such as clotrimazole, sulconizole, and ciclopirox, to name a few, are effective in most cases. Oral griseoful-vin suspension (Grifulvin) may be needed for more resistant cases. For a complete cure, treatment generally must be continued for several weeks, until repeat fungal cultures show no evidence of persistent infection. Stopping therapy too soon is one reason for rapid recurrence.

Tinea Capitis

In young children, fungal infections of the scalp, or *tinea capitis,* are a relatively common cause of hair loss, giving rise to hairless patches ranging from ½ inch to more than an inch in diameter. A number of fungi are capable of causing the problem, including some that can be transmitted from infected cats or dogs, as well as from infected humans.

Signs and symptoms vary depending on the specific infecting fungus. For example, one type causes redness, scaling, pustule formation, and hair breakage above the scalp surface. A second fungal invader mainly causes hair breakage close to the scalp, creating a dotlike look—a condition nicknamed *black-dot tinea capitis.* Finally, some children develop *kerions,* large, boggy, pus-filled swellings in the scalp covered by pustules and crusts.

Diagnosing tineas of the scalp may require microscopic and fungal culture examinations of scrapings from the scalp and hair. The Wood's ultraviolet light may also be helpful, fluorescing a yellowish green in the presence of certain fungi. Because of their inability to reach to the depth of the hair follicles, topical therapies are generally ineffective. Oral griseofulvin taken for six to twelve weeks, however, is curative in the vast majority of instances. In addition to griseofulvin, kerions may benefit from a three-week course of oral steroids to reduce inflammation. Finally, any household pets that may be sources of infection should be thoroughly examined and treated by a veterinarian.

10

BUGS AND OTHER PESTS

Just when you thought that allergens, bacteria, viruses, and fungi were more than enough for any child to contend with, you need to keep in mind the host of biting and stinging bugs and other nasty critters out there just waiting for their turn to cause problems. Particularly during warm weather, at the beach, in the park, or even in your own backyard, your child's delicate skin can become a favorite target for a wide array of attacking creatures. And biting and stinging are not necessarily all these little beasties do to their victims. Some may inject toxic chemicals, and others trigger allergic reactions. Still others can transmit serious infections, such as the much publicized Lyme disease.

Bug bites, stings, infestations, and related infections would require a huge book of their own. Only some of the more common and important conditions are discussed here, including assaults by several types of eight-legged creatures (arachnids) and a number of six-legged bugs (insects), together called *arthropods*.

ARACHNIDS

Scabies

Scabies is a disease, or, more precisely, an infestation, caused by the itch mite, *Sarcoptes scabiei*, a pinpoint-sized bug barely visible to the naked eye. This creature prefers to attack the thin-skinned regions of the body, which are relatively free from hair and oil glands. Individuals of any age, are affected, including infants, are potential targets. At present, scabies is epidemic in the United States, affecting millions of people. Because it is spread through intimate body contact, it is one of the more prevalent venereally transmissible diseases.

The female mite is the troublemaker, burrowing a home in her victim's skin that can range in size from ⅛ inch to several inches in length. Tiny, pimplelike spots and blisters or pustules appear shortly thereafter, as the organism begins to multiply and spread to other areas. Within four to six weeks, the rash becomes severely itchy, a condition believed to be an allergic reaction. Blistery lesions are more common in infants and young children and involve the face, head, and neck. But the rash may cover the entire body and can be particularly severe in infants, small children, and those with a history of atopic eczema (see Chapter 7). The palms of the hands and soles of the feet can also be involved. (In older children and adults, the rash more typically involves the groin, armpit, nipple, and belly button regions).

The itch of scabies is generally so intense that many burrows are destroyed by scratching. Scratch marks, eczema, crusts, and secondary infection become common complications. For reasons that remain unclear, some children develop *nodular scabies,* in which brownish red nodules form on the armpits, groin, buttocks, genital area, and shoulders. Finally, a less severe form of scabies can be transmitted from dogs infested with the canine scabies mite (mange). The fact that humans are not this creature's preferred host accounts for the mild, short-lived nature of this condition.

Unfortunately, unless your child's physician suspects the diagnosis, scabies may be missed in infants and young children. Scraping possible burrows in a search for the mite can be helpful, and occasionally a skin biopsy may be needed to confirm the diagnosis. A variety of treatments have proven successful, including the use of 6% precipitated sulfur in petroleum jelly, lindane lotion (Kwell, Scabene), and crotamiton lotion (Eurax). More recently, the FDA approved a permethrin compound, Elimite, for use in scabies. Its safety and efficacy record make it the current medication of choice for all age-groups.

Regardless of which agent is chosen, however, antiscabies medications work most effectively when left on overnight. To prevent Ping-Pong reinfections, all family members in close contact should be treated at the same time. In addition, bed sheets, pajamas, towels, linens, and such must be laundered in hot water to ensure the destruction of any living mites. However, overzealous scrubbing, washing, and bathing, which worsen dryness and increase itching, should be avoided. Unfortunately, itching often persists for days to weeks after all the mites have been destroyed, and oral antihistamines, topical antiitch medications, and topical steroid creams may be needed until the symptoms have entirely subsided.

Ticks

Found in grasses, shrubs, bushes, and vines, *ticks* may be conceived of as bigger mites. They are bloodsucking creatures who bury their heads in the victim's skin and take their meals from the superficial blood vessels. Bites are usually painless and may go unnoticed for days, until the surrounding areas swell and redden. If the tick is improperly removed, its mouth parts may become embedded and cause a nodule in the skin that may remain for weeks to years.

Lyme disease, named for the town in Connecticut where an epidemic outbreak was first researched, is a national and world-wide problem, seen in thirty-two states and on five continents. The disease is caused by the bacterium *Borrelia burgdorferi,* a relative of the syphilis organism, which is transmitted to humans through the bite of the pinhead-sized tick *Ixodes dammini,* the deer tick. At present, Lyme disease is America's number-one tick-borne infectious disease. Spring and summer are the prime times for outbreaks, and California, Connecticut, Massachusetts, Minnesota, New York, New Jersey, Rhode Island, and Wisconsin are notable hot spots.

The signs of Lyme disease include a peculiar skin rash known as *erythema chronicum migrans,* which begins sometime between two days and several weeks after the bite. The rash, which appears in about two-thirds of cases, starts as a small, reddish spot, then expands significantly as the causative bacteria spread beyond the site of the bite. The rash may vary in size from 2 to 3 inches to as much as 20 inches in diameter. In some cases, it can be intensely red, in others so faint as to be missed. At other times, the rash may have deeply red borders and a clear center or may assume a bull's-eye configuration. The thighs, groin, and armpits are favored locations.

Lyme disease may progress through three stages. In the first stage, the rash may be accompanied by fatigue, headache, fever, chills, and muscle aches. When the rash does not appear, these may be the only signs and symptoms of the disease. If left untreated, within weeks to months the disease may progress to the second stage, in which the heart and nervous system are attacked. The third stage, chronic arthritis, may begin a year or more later.

In the absence of the rash, diagnosing Lyme disease can be particularly difficult. To make matters worse, current diagnostic laboratory tests are notoriously unhelpful until about six weeks after the bite, when blood antibody levels to the infecting organism have risen sufficiently to be picked up. Treatment with oral penicillin or erythromycin in the early stages of the disease can prevent the later consequences. Intravenous antibiotic therapy may be needed for more advanced cases.

Prevention, of course, remains the best form of therapy for Lyme disease. Some recommendations include wearing shoes, socks, and long pants cinched at the ankles when outdoors in grassy and wooded areas and staying on paths rather than walking through tall bushes and grass. Light-colored clothing is preferable, so ticks can be more easily spotted. You should make it a habit to examine your child for ticks each night between mid-April and mid-September. Flea and tick collars are not particularly useful against the bearer of this disease, so check your pets, too. Tick repellents (Cutter and Off are two examples) for use on clothing and skin usually contain DEET (diethyl-meta-toluamide), which repels ticks but does *not* kill them. They are best used on clothing.

Spider Bites

There seems to be an almost limitless variety of spiders. However, only two, the black widow and the brown recluse, are responsible for all the serious bites in the United States. The female *black widow,* recognized by its jet black color and the red-orange hourglass marking on its rounded belly, bites only in self-defense. With its pincerlike teeth, the spider causes two pinpoint, burning or stinging, reddish swellings. Soon after, the bite area whitens and becomes surrounded by an intense, reddish halo that may grow to several inches in diameter. Within ten to sixty minutes, a severe, painful cramping occurs in the thighs, back, belly, and chest muscles, which worsens during the next three hours. Headaches, nausea, vomiting, fever, and conjunctivitis are common accompaniments.

The black widow's bite may be fatal in approximately 5 percent of children, but most, fortunately, recover completely in a few days, although residual problems may persist for several weeks. Treatment consists of specific antivenom therapy given intramuscularly and muscle relaxants, such as calcium gluconate, administered intravenously. Valium, for additional muscle relaxation, and pain medications such as morphine may also be required. Unfortunately, no effective spider repellents are currently available. Insecticides can be helpful in keeping the spider population down.

The *brown recluse spider,* recognized by the violin- or fiddle-shaped marking on its back, also bites only in self-defense. It is a little smaller than the black widow, measuring only 1 to 2 inches in diameter. Redness, swelling, itching, and stinging are common results of a brown recluse bite, but most bites are not serious. Nevertheless, children who have already become allergic and those exposed to an unusually large volume of venom may suffer severe reactions within forty-eight hours of a bite. The surrounding area becomes red and swollen and its center bluish or purple and pus filled; a gangrenelike breakdown of the skin soon follows. These changes can be accompanied by nausea, vomiting, headaches, muscle aches, and fever.

Treatment consists of bed rest, elevation of the affected limb, compresses, ice packs, and oral antibiotics and oral steroids when appropriate. Antivenom therapy and the use of a special sulfur-containing antibiotic, Avlosulfone (dapsone), have also been effective in reducing skin breakdown. Depending on the extent of damage, skin grafting may be needed to repair the damaged area.

Lice

Three kinds of *lice* have plagued humankind since time immemorial: *Pediculus capitis,* the head louse; *Pediculus corporis,* the body louse; and *Phthirus pubis,* the pubic (crab) louse, which is not common to young children. In all three cases, adult lice hatch from nits, which are grayish to yellowish white, pinhead-sized eggs. Nits attach themselves to scalp hair in head louse infestation, to the seams of clothing or bedding in body louse infestation, and in adults to the pubic hairs and eyelashes in pubic louse infestation. Eggs reach maturity in approximately two weeks. Unlike dandruff particles, with which they are often confused, nits are tightly anchored to the hair shaft and cannot be easily dislodged.

Passed readily from one child to another, *head lice* infestation is common among school-age children. Girls appear particularly prone to the problem, perhaps because of their longer hairstyles. Sharing hats, combs, hairbrushes, and towels contributes to the spread. You should carefully examine for nits attached to the hair, especially above the nape of the neck and above the ears.

Body lice live in clothing and bedding and attack the human host only for feeding, leaving pinpoint, reddish marks, pimples, or hives. As a rule, itching is so intense that scratch marks can eventually cover practically the entire body; crusting and secondary infection are common. You should look for adult lice and nits in the seams of clothing or bedding.

Although closely related to the other two, the *crab louse* is technically a different species. Infestation, most often found in sexually active young adults, is uncommon in children and can usually be traced to contact with an infested adult, generally the mother.

In any form of louse infestation, discovering adult lice or nits confirms the diagnosis. A Wood's ultraviolet light examination by your doctor can be helpful, because nits will fluoresce a pearly color under such light, whereas dandruff and lint will not. Occasionally, microscopic examination of the nits is needed for confirmation.

Because the body louse lives in clothing or bedding, treating the infestation is simply a matter of hot-water laundering, boiling, or dry-cleaning all intimate laundry to kill the adult lice and nits. Head lice infestation is treated by shampooing with lindane shampoo (Kwell, Scabene) or by applying lindane lotion and leaving it on overnight. Alternative therapies include pyrethrins (for instance, **RID**, A-200), or Nix (permethrin). If necessary, treatment can be repeated in a week. To prevent reinfestation, simultaneously treating family and all close contacts is advisable.

It is important to know that killing the nits in this way will not necessarily dislodge them from the hair shafts. To do this, soak your child's hair with plain white vinegar for about an hour. The acetic acid in vinegar disrupts the bonds between the eggs and the hair shafts. The nits can then be more easily removed with tweezers or a fine-tooth comb. For more information about these conditions, or for ways to increase community awareness of the louse problem, contact the National Pediculosis Association, P.O. Box 149, Newton, MA 02161.

Fleas

Fleas are true nuisances, and people are susceptible to attack not only by fleas from humans but by cat and dog fleas as well. Like body lice, fleas spend most of their lives away from their host animal, attacking only periodically to feed. Bites generally appear in groups or clusters on the arms, forearms, waist, buttocks, thighs, and lower legs (especially near the ankles). Individual bites may appear pimple- or hivelike and possess pinpoint-sized, bloody centers. Itching can be intense.

Topical corticosteroids usually suffice to relieve itching. Occasionally oral antihistamines may be needed. Because fleas can remain alive for from several weeks to a year without feeding, to eradicate the problem completely the source of the infestation must be located and treated. Carpets, furniture stuffing, bedding, baseboards, and crevices where fleas typically take up residence should be sprayed with pyrethrin (**RID**), or commercial insecticides. Vigorous vacuuming should follow to remove eggs and cocoons. Professional exterminators may also be needed. Of course, infested pets must be treated according to the instructions of your veterinarian. (Warning: Flea collars are not useful once fleas have infested the home and should not be relied on.)

Bedbugs

The feeding habits of *bedbugs* are similar to those of fleas and body lice; they spend most of their time away from their host animal, living in cracks and crevices in furniture and other household structures. They skulk out at night only to feed.

The common bedbug is about ¼ inch long, flat, oval, and reddish brown. It attacks at night while its victim is asleep in bed, hence its name. The bite is usually painless and seldom awakens its victim. Bedbug bites closely resemble those of fleas, although, by contrast, they are generally located on exposed areas: the face, neck, arms, and hands. One or more bites may be present.

Symptomatic treatment and eradication measures are identical to those described for fleas. Like fleas, bedbugs have been known to survive up to a year without feeding. Unfortunately, exterminating them can be difficult, even for professionals.

INSECTS

Hymenoptera Stings

Bees, wasps, hornets, and yellow jackets belong to a group of stinging insects known as *Hymenoptera* (insects with membraneous wings). Although not a flying insect, the ferocious fire ant, prevalent in the South, is also a part of this group. All possess large, venom-producing glands at the tip of the abdomen. In general, Hymenoptera sting only when frightened or provoked. If the present rate of fatalities from bee stings continues, more people will die from them than from all other insect attacks combined.

Individual reactions to stings can run the gamut from mild local eruptions to severe, life-threatening episodes. Most stings cause only redness, mild swelling, itching, or pain that last for a few hours and subside on their own. Mild reactions are not believed to be allergic. However, more extensive local reactions, progressing to involve an entire limb, for example, are felt to be allergy related, as are severe systemic reactions. In such cases, severe swelling may be accompanied by nausea, vomiting, dizziness, and wheezing. In extreme cases, the child may suffer a precipitous drop in blood pressure and respiratory failure, necessitating immediate emergency medical care.

First aid for simple Hymenoptera stings involves scraping the skin to remove the stinger and attached venom sac, if still present, and applying ice. Your child's doctor may also prescribe a topical corticosteroid cream and oral antihistamine. Oral steroids may be needed for more extensive local reactions. Violent reactions necessitate the immediate administration of epinephrine (adrenaline) and may also call for the use of blood pressure–elevating medications and respiratory assistance.

In warm weather, preventive measures for the outdoors include not wearing brightly colored clothing, flowery prints, or scented lotions, or consuming sweets, syrupy drinks, or sodas. Commercial insect repellents unfortunately are ineffective and should not be relied on. Parents, especially of children known to be hypersensitive to stings, should carry commercial emergency kits containing antihistamine tablets, a tourniquet, syringe, and epinephrine ampules at all times and should be thoroughly familiar with their proper use.

Any child who has experienced a violent reaction to Hymenoptera stings should be evaluated by a pediatric allergist. Intradermal skin tests and a special blood test known as the RAST (radioallergosorbent test) may be used to determine specific allergies to Hymenoptera venom and venom components. Desensitization shots (similar to the kind used for hay fever sufferers) employing venom sac contents have proven successful in reducing the risk of potentially life-threatening reactions from about 60 percent to 5 percent. These shots are given about twice weekly for the first three months; to ensure maximal immunity, periodic booster shots are usually continued for about five years. Because some risk remains despite this therapy, it is still advisable to carry an emergency kit.

Mosquitoes, Biting Flies, and Gnats

Mosquitoes, biting flies, and *gnats* are all related, and much of what is said about mosquitoes applies to the other two. All of us, at one time or another, have been bitten by a mosquito, and the typical itchy, pale, hivelike bite is easily recognizable. An ordinary bite lasts about a day. In sensitized children, however, bites can produce large hives and severe itching that may last for several days.

Diagnosing mosquito bites generally presents no problem, and treatment other than ice packs for ordinary bites is seldom needed. More extensive local reactions may be treated as described for Hymenoptera stings (see page 130). Prevention consists of avoiding brightly colored or floral-patterned clothing (stick with white, green, or khaki) and scented products or lotions (one more reason to use hypoallergenic moisturizers and sunscreens; see Chapters 1 and 2). DEET-containing insect repellents, such as Cutter and Off, are quite effective and can be safely used on children over one year of age.

Caterpillars

Caterpillars are at an intermediate stage in the life cycle of moths and butterflies. Certain kinds of moths and caterpillars possess venom glands at the bases of their hairs; these hairs can become detached and cause problems to humans by either direct or airborne contact. Reactions range from itching, burning, or stinging to measleslike spots, hives, small blisters, and tiny ulcerations at the points of contact. Airborne reactions tend to be more widespread, giving rise to eye irritations, fever, numbness, muscle pains, and lymph gland enlargement. Symptoms may persist for two weeks.

Your child's doctor can confirm the diagnosis of caterpillar dermatitis by scraping the skin and examining the sample under a microscope for the presence of caterpillar hairs. Ice packs can help decrease swelling and discomfort, and adhesive or cellophane tape placed over the irritated area, then gently lifted off, may help remove any embedded spines or hairs. Oral antihistamines and topical steroids may also be helpful. Systemic steroids may be prescribed for more severe reactions.

JELLYFISH

Even the harmless-looking, transparent glob of a *jellyfish* can cause skin problems, and jellyfish stings are by no means uncommon in ocean bathers. Reactions, called *jellyfish dermatosis,* may be either irritant or allergic and can range from very mild stinging and burning to severe hives and even shock. Although the *Portuguese man-of-war* is probably the best-known cause of severe jellyfish reactions, other jellyfish are also capable of illiciting these reactions.

Whole jellyfish need not be present to cause problems. They are capable of releasing barbed, toxin-containing, cystlike structures into the water that can affect swimmers nearby without direct contact. In addition, severe storms may detach tentacles from jellyfish that retain their capacity to cause reactions even months later. These are believed to be the cause of the epidemics of itching and rashes often observed by lifeguards after storms. Unaware that they have been stung, swimmers may inadvertently trigger a reaction by rubbing embedded jellyfish cysts, releasing their toxin.

The most common form of eruption is a line-shaped, poison ivy–like rash that appears within minutes of direct contact with the jellyfish or the detached cysts or tentacles. Less often, the rash can occur as many as five days later.

Treatment must be directed at preventing the "firing" of unruptured cysts. To this end, vinegar soaks or sprays may be helpful. Applying a paste of water and a meat tenderizer (for example, Adolph's) that contains a protein-denaturing enzyme may also be tried to deactivate the venom. Any jellyfish parts remaining stuck to the skin must be manually removed. Systemic painkillers are sometimes needed for a few days.

PAPULAR URTICARIA

I couldn't conclude this chapter on nasty critters without a description of *papular urticaria,* an allergic condition linked to the bites of a variety of insects, including fleas, bedbugs, and mosquitoes. It is not surprising that this problem is seasonal, usually occurring during spring and summer, the height of the bug season.

Generally affecting children between the ages of two and seven, papular urticaria is marked by the appearance of waves of hivelike pimples ranging from ⅛ to ½ inches in diameter; some possess a central prick mark, the site of the bite. Although the exposed areas of the face, neck, chest, backs of thighs, and buttocks are the most common locations, the entire body may be affected. The typically widespread nature of the rash is believed to be an allergic reaction to several bites, not the result of numerous bites all over. Individual spots may persist from two to ten days, and occasionally the reaction lingers well beyond the end of the bug season. Recurrences are not uncommon, especially in children with a personal or family history of atopy (asthma, hay fever, and eczema).

A history of exaggerated sensitivity to insect bites and a personal or family history of atopy help establish the diagnosis of papular urticaria. Treatment includes oral antihistamines and topical and systemic steroids. Parents should see to it that the measures described on page 130 for prevention and avoidance of insect bites be strictly followed.

11

HAIR AND NAIL PROBLEMS

The hair and nails of children are as vulnerable to problems as their skin. Happily, many of these conditions require of parents only reassurance and a bit of patience, and others little more than simple at-home measures. Although more complex problems generally necessitate professional consultation and care, safe and effective treatments are currently available for most childhood hair and nail disorders.

Diseases of either the hair or the nails are basically of two kinds, those that exclusively affect the hair or nails and those in which the problems are part of more widespread skin conditions, such as seborrheic dermatitis or psoriasis. The topic of hair and nail conditions is extensive and would require a book in itself. Only some of the more important problems in infants and young children are discussed in this chapter.

NORMAL HAIR

Hair is basically a fabriclike material composed of *nonliving* protein. This point bears emphasis because shampoo and hair care product advertisers continue to hype formulas purported to "bring back life to hair" or to make it "come alive." This is nothing short of nonsense. You can no more make your hair come back to life than you can bring life back to the fibers in your sweater.

Hairs grow from *follicles*, which are found just about everywhere on the body except the palms of the hands, soles of the feet, sides of the fingers and toes, lips, and the shaft of the penis. At the base of each follicle is a *hair bulb,* or *root,* the only truly living and regenerating area of the hair-making machinery. On average, the normal human scalp contains about 100,000 hairs, blondes having slightly more and redheads slightly fewer.

In humans, hair grows in several stages. You need only acquaint yourself with two: the *anagen* (or growing) phase, which lasts about three years, and the *telogen* (or resting) phase, which lasts about three weeks. At the end of each complete cycle, new anagen hairs push out old telogen hairs and the cycle begins again. At any time, approximately 80 percent of human hairs are in the growing phase and 15 percent in the resting phase. In general, scalp hairs grow slightly less than ½ inch each month.

HAIR PROBLEMS

Congenital Hypertrichosis

In the womb, hair development begins between the eighth and twelfth weeks of life and continues through pregnancy. Before birth, the infant's entire body and face are covered with a dense growth of fine, light-colored hairs, known as *lanugo hairs.* Normally, these hairs are shed by the end of the seventh or eighth month of fetal life. Preemies, born before shedding can occur, may enter the world covered with lanugo hairs, a condition doctors refer to as *congenital hypertrichosis.* The name simply means "excessive hairiness at birth." To uninitiated parents, seeing their newborn covered with hair can be distressing. But patience is the only therapy needed; lanugo hairs are shed during the first six months of life and replaced by normal hair with normal distribution.

Neonatal (Newborn) Hair

Some parents also worry needlessly about what are simply normal variations in the pattern of hair distribution and shedding in full-term babies. Although it may be cosmetically distressing, newborns' hairlines can extend across their foreheads, along their temples, and even down to their eyebrows. Reassurance is the only therapy needed here, too, because the problem generally lasts only a few weeks, until the unwanted hairs are shed naturally.

Too little hair can also needlessly raise parental anxiety. Under ordinary circumstances, at birth most hairs are in the growing phase. Many are shifted shortly thereafter into the resting phase and extruded within the first four months of life. This process of hair loss and replacement is usually gradual and imperceptible. Sometimes, however, normal hair loss can occur so rapidly that complete balding results. Once again, there is no real need to worry. Complete regrowth takes place within six months.

Telogen Effluvium (Stress-induced Hair Loss)

On average, a healthy scalp loses between fifty and one hundred resting hairs every day, each of which is simultaneously replaced by a new, growing hair. Periods of intense emotional or physical stress, however, can upset this pattern and lead to a distressing, significant loss of hair known as *telogen effluvium*. Disruptive stresses include episodes of high fevers, severe illness, surgery, injury, and emotional trauma. This condition is by far the most common cause of hair loss in children (and second only to hereditary hair loss in adults).

Telogen effluvium generally begins within one to four months after a stressful episode and continues for several months. How many hair follicles are affected depends on the child and the duration and severity of the triggering stress. In extreme cases, batches of hairs will be found each morning on the pillow and in the hairbrush. If the process continues, scalp areas may begin showing. Between 25,000 and 40,000 hairs must be lost for balding to become apparent.

Diagnosing telogen hair loss rests on linking the sudden loss to a recent stress. To confirm the clinical impression, your child's dermatologist may recommend that you make a weekly hair collection for several weeks so that he or she can more accurately assess the rate of loss. On average, loss of more than one hundred hairs per day is highly supportive of the diagnosis. The doctor may also perform a hair pluck test. For this, a small clump of hairs is grasped in a clamp and pulled free. By examining the hairs under a hand lens or microscope, the physician can compare the ratio of anagen to telogen hairs. If the proportion of telogen hairs exceeds 25 percent (remember, normal is 15 percent), the diagnosis is confirmed.

Because no effective therapies are currently available for telogen effluvium, you'll find it comforting that spontaneous regrowth is the rule, usually within six months after the stress has abated. Naturally, continued illness or repeated episodes of the triggering stress can delay recovery.

Alopecia Areata

Alopecia areata is a common condition in which oval or round bald spots suddenly appear. Although its precise cause remains unknown, alopecia areata is believed to be an autoimmune disease—a condition in which the body's natural germ-fighting system somehow goes awry and mistakenly attacks the hair follicles. A family history of the disorder is present in as many as 20 percent of cases.

The onset of the disorder may occur overnight or more gradually, over one to three weeks. The scalp is the most frequent site of attack, but any hair-bearing area of the body can be involved. One or more completely hairless, smooth, and ivory patches may be present, ranging from 1 inch to 5 or more inches in diameter. At the edge of these patches, there may be short hairs resembling exclamation marks. These are highly characteristic of alopecia areata and are helpful for diagnosing the condition. New bald patches may appear for several months. *Ophiasis* is the special name given to alopecia areata when it occasionally occurs as a broad bald patch directly over an ear.

In about 5 percent of children, alopecia areata progresses slowly to *alopecia totalis,* the complete loss of all scalp hair. A far smaller percentage go on to lose all body hair, including the eyebrows and eyelashes, a problem termed *alopecia universalis.* Finally, about 20 percent of children with alopecia areata, for reasons that are unclear, simultaneously develop obvious pitting of the fingernails.

Diagnosing alopecia areata seldom presents a problem. When there is some question, however, a biopsy can be helpful. Unhappily, the earlier the onset of the disorder and the more severe or extensive the episode, the poorer the outcome for complete regrowth. In cases of limited involvement, the outlook is excellent in 95 percent of children, and regrowth usually takes between four and forty weeks from the time of onset. Future episodes are likely, however, in approximately one-third of these children.

Topical corticosteroids remain the mainstay of therapy for this condition in children. A high-potency topical steroid may be applied twice daily directly to the hairless patch or placed under occlusion (shower cap, Actiderm dressing, or Saran Wrap taped in place) to increase its absorption and efficacy. Intralesional injections of corticosteroids, administered about once a month, are reserved for more resistant cases. Although it is believed that steroids hasten regrowth, there is no proof that they alter the overall outcome in any way. Oral steroids are rarely prescribed, except in the most severe cases.

A variety of other topical irritants and allergens, including poison ivy resin, anthralin dinitrochlorobenzene (DNCB), and squaric acid dibutyl ester have all been used through the years with variable success to stimulate hair regrowth. No one knows for sure how they work. Topical minoxidil lotion (Rogaine), currently used to treat certain types of male pattern baldness, has also demonstrated some success. For the best care, a dermatologist experienced in dealing with alopecia areata in children should be consulted. For more information, you may contact the National Alopecia Areata Foundation, 714 C Street, Suite 216, San Rafael, CA 94901.

Traction Alopecia

If they are worn for prolonged periods, certain hairstyles that place hair under sustained tension can lead to hair shaft weakening, breakage, and permanent hair loss, resulting in a condition aptly known as *traction alopecia*. Ponytails, for example, can cause hair loss at the sides of the scalp, the points of maximum stress from this style. Rollers, by contrast, tend to cause stress at the front center of the scalp. And tight braids or cornrows, hairstyles popular with black children, may produce diffuse hair loss throughout the scalp. Fortunately, if the culprit style is changed before permanent damage has occurred to the hair roots, the process is entirely reversible. No other therapies are usually necessary.

Trichotillomania (Hair-pulling Tics)

Trichotillomania refers to the conscious or subconscious habit of pulling, rubbing, twirling, or tugging on the hair, which leads to hair breakage and partial hair loss. Occasionally, the eyebrows and eyelashes are also involved. This practice can be likened to nail biting. Seen slightly more frequently in girls, trichotillomania generally affects children between the ages of four and ten.

The front or side of the scalp is most often affected, usually on the side opposite the dominant hand. Although only one site is generally involved, more may be present. Typically, these sites are irregular in outline and composed of short, stubbly, or broken hairs. Scratch marks may also be seen.

Diagnosing trichotillomania usually presents little difficulty, especially if the child is caught manipulating the hair. When doubt exists, however, a biopsy may be helpful. Haranguing the child to stop the habit is generally unsuccessful, although distracting him with other activities may sometimes work. An understanding dermatologist who offers encouragement and prescribes a gentle placebo shampoo or lotion is more likely to meet success.

Happily, in many cases complete hair regrowth can be expected to occur spontaneously if the process has not gone on so long that hair follicles have become permanently destroyed. Treatment is more challenging and less rewarding, however, when neither the child nor the parents seem aware of the habit or simply deny it.

Trichorrhexis Nodosa

Resulting most often from too vigorous toweling, brushing, or combing, or from overexposure to sun and saltwater, *trichorrhexis nodosa* is the most common acquired abnormality of the hair shaft. In this condition, the child's hair becomes dry, lusterless, and stubbly. To the naked eye, affected hairs appear to have small, knoblike bumps (or nodes) somewhere along their length. Under the microscope, however, each hair, which is actually partially fractured, resembles two brooms or brushes with their straw ends pushed together. The hair may eventually return to normal if gentle hair care practices are instituted right away; the use of conditioners can also sometimes be helpful. Regrowth is slow and may take from several months to several years.

NORMAL NAILS

Like hair, nails are composed of nonliving protein, and no "miracle" cosmetics, or medications for that matter, can bring them back to life. The living and growing area of the nail, equivalent to the hair root, is located directly under the skin at the base of the nail and is called the *nail matrix*. The *lunula*, the whitish area at the base of the nail, is the only visible portion of the growing area. The cuticle, directly above it, is a small extension of skin bridging the nail to the rest of the skin on the fingers and toes. Infections or other diseases that affect the matrix can permanently distort the nail or disrupt its growth entirely. On average, fingernails grow approximately ¼ inch per month.

At birth, normal nails are smooth, thin, flat, flexible, and transparent. Occasionally, the nails of the big toes may be spoon shaped, and the lunula may not be visible in all nails. A large percentage of normal newborns possess depressions across their fingernails, known as *Beau's lines*. Their cause in normal infants is not known, although in older children they can result from prior nail injury or infection. Beau's lines may be first noticed at about four weeks of age. They grow out completely by about fourteen weeks. No treatment is necessary.

NAIL PROBLEMS

Subungual Hematoma

Subungual hematoma literally means "accumulation of blood under the nail." Resulting from injuries such as slamming the fingertip with a hammer or other heavy object or catching a finger in a door, subungual hematomas are probably the most common type of injury to the nail. When the trauma is to the growing area, rather than to the nail itself, blood may not appear for two to three days. Thereafter, it will continue to move forward slowly as the nail grows out. Usually no treatment other than reassurance is necessary.

If the injury is directly to the nail plate, however, hemorrhage below the nail usually becomes apparent immediately. As pressure rises from blood accumulating under the nail, pain may become intense. Treatment consists of relieving the pressure by piercing a hole through the nail, with either a cautery device or a paper clip heated to red hot in a flame. You may cringe at the thought, but the procedure is actually quite painless, and anesthesia is not necessary; with the evacuation of the blood, welcome pain relief is immediate. If the procedure is not performed soon enough, partial, although temporary, shedding of the nail may occur during the next several weeks.

Nail and Cuticle Biting

Nail biting and *cuticle biting* are common habits that can cause considerable damage to the nail as well as the surrounding tissue. Stress is believed to play a major role in these habits.

Diagnosing bitten nails usually presents little difficulty, although occasionally a child may deny the habit. Contrary to a popular misconception, bitten nails actually grow slightly faster than normal; nevertheless, because of the continual biting, they are usually very short and irregular.

Nail and cuticle biters spend a great deal of time gnawing off tiny spicules, nail or cuticle fragments, formed from earlier biting sessions. Some children attack only one nail, leaving the others alone. Much less commonly, all the nails, or all except one, may be ravaged. Deformed nails, raggedness, infection, hangnails, and warts are common complications of nail biting. Giving up the habit is the obvious cure for the problem; unfortunately, this is often difficult to accomplish. Keeping the nails coated with bitter-tasting preparations designed to discourage biting is occasionally effective in helping break the habit.

Hangnails

Hangnails, which develop very commonly in nail biters, are not really nails at all. Instead, they are fleshy bits of skin that have split away from the nail folds, the skin around the sides of the nail. Hangnails can also result from any kind of injury to the area. Often extending deep into the skin, hangnails can be exceedingly painful and pave the way for secondary infection. Resist the temptation to pull them off. Hangnails are best treated by cutting off the flap of flesh at its base with a clipper or sharp-pointed scissors.

Paronychia

A *paronychia* is literally an infection around a nail. In this condition, the skin directly behind the cuticles or around the nail folds becomes tender, swollen, red, and infected. Pus may be visible to the side of the nail and can often be expressed, or squeezed out. The cuticle is frequently broken or entirely absent. Depending on how long the problem has been present, the nail plate may show the horizontal, white, rippled marks called Beau's lines. In more protracted cases, especially those affecting the growing areas, the nails may thicken, become yellowish white, and crumble.

Persistent wetness and trauma to the nail folds predisposes the nails to paronychias by disrupting the normal skin barrier to infection. Bacteria, such as *Staphylococcus aureus* and streptococcus or the yeast organism, *Candida (Monilia),* are the most common causes of infectious paronychias. Children who are thumb suckers, nail biters, or nail or cuticle pickers are particularly prone to this condition.

Diagnosing paronychia is generally not difficult, although bacterial and fungal microscopic examinations and cultures may be needed to pinpoint the causative organism. Depending on the cause, treatment may consist of oral or topical antibiotics or antifungal agents. Thumb sucking or other disruptive nail habits that can damage nails should be discouraged. For small children, a white cotton sock can be placed over the involved hand to prevent sucking during sleep.

12

BLOOD VESSEL BIRTHMARKS

Few skin problems can be more upsetting and frightening to new parents than a disfiguring *blood vessel beauty mark* prominently located on the face of their newborn. But, alarming though they may be, the majority of these marks shrink and disappear completely on their own in a few years. Even when they don't, a variety of successful techniques are available for significantly correcting most such defects and restoring baby-beautiful skin.

Blood vessel beauty marks, correctly known as *hemangiomas,* are sometimes also referred to as *vascular birthmarks* or *vascular nevi.* Because they are filled with blood, most hemangiomas appear red or reddish purple. If salmon patches are included with them (see Chapter 4), blood vessel beauty marks make up the largest single group of skin growths in infancy and childhood.

Affecting as many as 10 percent of babies, hemangiomas may develop as a result of hereditary factors or from subtle developmental abnormalities during intrauterine development. They may either be present at birth or develop shortly afterward. Girls are affected about twice as often as boys.

There are three main types of hemangiomas: port wine stain, strawberry hemangioma, and cavernous hemangioma. Each may appear anywhere on the skin or the mucous membranes of the nose, mouth, anus, or vagina. Rarely, they may develop in internal organs or within the skull bones, where they are discovered by special tests. Many are quite small, although some hemangiomas grow to involve an entire arm or leg. When they involve the face, they can pose a significant cosmetic problem and can become the source of much psychological distress to parents and to older children. Happily, the vast majority of hemangiomas disappear spontaneously and require no treatment other than a tincture of time and patience.

PORT WINE STAINS

The *port wine stain,* also called *nevus flammeus,* is by far the most common of the three types of blood vessel beauty marks. Although they may appear on the arms, legs, chest, and back, port wine stains most frequently affect the neck and face. Fortunately, many occur on the back of the scalp or nape of the neck and are hidden by hair. Red, purple, or bluish purple in color, port wine stains range from as small as a coin to large enough to cover half the face or even half the body.

At birth, port wine stains are typically smooth and flat. Later in life, however, they can thicken, darken, and become bumpy. Occasionally, especially when they involve the mouth, bleeding (sometimes heavy) may occur after injury.

A recent study in England of persons with disfiguring port wine stains underscored the psychological effects of this condition. Anxiety, depression, lack of self-esteem, feelings of sexual unattractiveness, and withdrawal from social situations were common complaints among people with this abnormality. The study also found that older individuals showed no lessening of concern about their appearance. To prevent such difficulties, early treatment is advisable.

Diagnosing port wine stains is seldom the problem that treating them has been until recently. In the past, X-ray therapy, skin grafting, dermabrasion (skin sanding), cryotherapy, and tattooing have all been tried with limited success. These treatments now have largely been abandoned. For many years, only special masking cosmetics permitted people with disfiguring vascular birthmarks to feel more confident in their appearance and regain their self-esteem. Covermark (1 Anderson Avenue, Moonachie, NJ 07074), Esteem (P.O. Box 5288, FDR Station, New York, NY 10022), and Dermablend (P.O. Box 3008, Lakewood, NJ 08701) are well-known manufacturers of these types of cosmetics and may be contacted directly for further information. Specially formulated, these masking cosmetics all are water-fast (staying on even after chlorine swimming) and capable of covering even deeply pigmented areas. On the down side, they are expensive, require about fifteen minutes to apply and to remove, and must be purchased either in special outlets or at large department stores. Nevertheless, for many people they make a normal life possible.

Recently, however, lasers have revolutionized the treatment of certain vascular birthmarks. Several types of lasers are being used with impressive results. For larger, deeper vessels, the continuous-wave, argon laser is frequently employed, and for smaller, finer vessels, the flash lamp–pumped dye laser is used. In either case, laser beams penetrate the skin and selectively strike the oxygen-carrying hemoglobin pigment in the red blood corpuscles, ultimately leading to irritation of the blood vessel walls and sealing of the unwanted vessels. In many cases, complete clearing or significant lightening is achieved after only a few treatments, generally about six. Because these lasers spare the overlying skin, scarring seldom results. Moreover, because laser therapy is relatively painless and requires no postoperative care, it is particularly well suited for children. Oral sedation before the procedure is usually advisable.

For more information, you may contact the National Congenital Port Wine Stain Foundation, 125 East Sixty-third Street, New York, NY 10021.

STRAWBERRY HEMANGIOMAS

Strawberry hemangiomas, also known as *capillary hemangiomas,* are not nearly as common as port wine stains. Projecting above the skin, these growths, which get their name from their striking surface resemblance to ripe strawberries, are typically red, spongy, and sharply demarcated from the surrounding normal skin. One or more of these hemangiomas may develop and may range from a few inches in diameter to large enough to encompass an entire arm or leg. The majority, however, tend to be small. Like port wine stains, strawberry hemangiomas can occur anywhere on the body, including the mucous membranes. They may be present at birth or develop within the first six months of life.

Strawberry birthmarks follow a fairly predictable pattern of growth and development. During the first few months, there is a rapid-growth phase in which they may increase to several times their original size. In some cases, this phase may last as long as eighteen months. In the second stage, a resting phase, the lesion may persist unchanged for several months. Finally, under ordinary circumstances, the birthmark begins to regress (shrink) spontaneously. Regression usually takes between two and six years. Fifty percent of children with these birthmarks show complete clearing by age five; 70 percent by age 7. In all, only 6 percent will require treatment.

In most cases, strawberry birthmarks leave little if any scarring after spontaneous clearing. And even those that do not completely clear will usually not cause much cosmetic concern. Finally, although a large strawberry birthmark may be alarming to parents, there appears to be no direct relationship between a lesion's size and its chances for complete spontaneous recovery.

Diagnosing strawberry hemangiomas is not difficult. Treatment should be considered only when the size or location of the mark impinges on vital structures or interferes with normal functioning, such as may occur with a growth on the foot, near the eye, or around the vagina. Other reasons for treatment include ulcer formation, hemorrhage, infection, or sudden, rapid enlargement.

When administered during the growth phase, oral and intralesional corticosteroids sometimes halt the progression of these hemangiomas and stimulate resolution. Repeated courses of treatment are occasionally necessary. Cryotherapy, surgical excision, and radiation therapy may also be useful, although radiotherapy is of no benefit in hemangiomas that have not shown any spontaneous shrinkage in seven years. Lasers, too, may be used, however, because of the thickness of these lesions, the results are generally less impressive than those obtained in the treatment of port wine stains.

A final word of caution: It has been repeatedly demonstrated that overall cosmetic results are better when nature takes care of this problem without any medical interference. The majority of strawberry hemangiomas, regardless of how alarming their initial appearance, will regress with time, and most physicians advise a waiting period of about four years, during which those hemangiomas inclined to shrink spontaneously will likely have done so. Although this time span can be painfully difficult for parents of children with unsightly hemangiomas, waiting remains, in most instances, the best course of action.

CAVERNOUS HEMANGIOMAS

Cavernous hemangiomas are similar to strawberry hemangiomas except that the blood vessels composing them are usually larger and more deeply situated. Although they may involve any location, cavernous hemangiomas favor the head and neck. Generally bluish red masses, they occasionally are so deep that the overlying skin appears essentially normal except for a trace of blue discoloration.

As a rule, cavernous hemangiomas are present at birth and grow rapidly during the first six to twelve months. Most average 1 to 2 inches in diameter; however, some may grow as large as 10 inches. Sometimes, a cavernous hemangioma is superimposed on a strawberry hemangioma.

The progression of these hemangiomas parallels that of strawberry birthmarks, the vast majority shrinking and disappearing entirely within a few years of development. Likewise, the reason for immediate treatment such as was mentioned on page 151 is the same, namely, interference with vital structures. Unfortunately, the ultimate cosmetic result may not always be as satisfactory as that seen with strawberry marks. Although the blood vessels in cavernous hemangiomas may shrink and disappear, the overlying skin typically persists as a soft outpouching. But again, waiting patiently several years for maximal improvement is still considered the best course of action. The surface outpouching may be surgically corrected, if necessary, at a later date.

PYOGENIC GRANULOMA

Although technically not a birthmark, the relatively common blood vessel overgrowth *pyogenic granuloma* bears a close physical resemblance to beauty marks. And, although the medical name implies bacterial infection and inflammation, neither process is really believed to play a role in this condition. Prior injury, however, may be an initiating factor, because these fragile, red to reddish brown nodules often occur on sites subject to trauma (fingers, face, forearms, and occasionally the oral mucous membranes). Usually only one nodule develops, normally measuring between ¼ inch and 1 inch in diameter. Because pyogenic granulomas possess a dense network of small blood vessels and are typically fragile, episodes of alarming bleeding are a common complaint.

Diagnosis is usually no problem, although a confirmatory biopsy is advisable in most cases. These lesions may be treated by a variety of destructive measures, including simple excision, cryosurgery, and electrosurgery, with excellent cosmetic results. Unfortunately, recurrences following any of these methods are not uncommon and require further treatment.

13

SERIOUS OR LIFE-THREATENING SKIN CONDITIONS

As you have seen in the previous chapters, most common skin conditions occurring in infancy and childhood are little more than temporary nuisances, regardless of how alarming they may appear. Many disappear spontaneously, others require only simple medical or surgical therapy. This chapter, however, covers several serious or potentially serious conditions that demand early recognition and close, specialized follow-up care to prevent or minimize physical and psychological complications and improve your child's quality of life. Despite the gravity of these conditions, and the current lack of cures for some, the pace at which medical research has been progressing in the past few years should give parents encouragement and hope that tomorrow will bring more effective treatments and cures.

CONGENITAL NEVI (TRUE BIRTHMARKS)

People frequently refer to ordinary moles as "birthmarks," even when they are aware that most moles actually developed some-time during childhood or adolescence. Strictly speaking, however, *congenital* pigmented moles (nevi) are those present *at the time of birth.* And this distinction is more than academic. When larger than approximately ⅗ inch in diameter, true congenital moles are believed to increase the individual's risk of developing *malignant melanoma,* a potentially life-threatening form of skin cancer.

Small congenital moles are generally flat and tan or pale brown; they initially resemble café au lait spots (see Chapter 5). Later, they elevate and become hairy. Giant congenital nevi, by contrast, are typically warty surfaced and have irregular borders. They vary from dark brown to jet black, and nearly all have hair growing from them. As the infant grows, the nevi generally become darker, thicker, rougher surfaced, and even nodular. They can often cover much of the scalp, face, trunk, arms, and legs and are frequently named "coat-sleeve," "bathing trunk," "stocking," or "capelike" nevi, depending on their location. As a rule, the distribution of these nevi parallels the course of underlying nerves.

Although there is no consensus on the precise risk imposed by congenital moles smaller than ⅗ inch, the larger ones, especially those covering much of the trunk or extremities, are estimated to have a chance of turning malignant between 2 and 40 percent. Warning signs include rapid growth, ulceration, crusting, bleeding, and changes in color (lightening or darkening of all or part of the growth).

Early treatment is especially important for large congenital moles, because the risk of malignancy increases with a child's age, and the highest risk of progression and metastasis (spread to other organs) occurs before the age of ten. Depending on size and location, larger congenital moles often necessitate several surgical removal procedures followed by skin grafting. In selected cases, dermabrasion (skin sanding) has been tried and, more recently, laser vaporization. The advantages of these methods are that large areas can be treated all at once, and no grafting is required. Neither of these procedures, however, goes deep enough to root out all the congenital nevus cells, which typically extend down the hair follicles. In general, giant congenital nevi carry a poor prognosis for the individual's survival.

By contrast, simple surgical excision is ideal for smaller lesions, and, when complete removal is possible, the outcome is uniformly excellent. Although the question of how small a congenital nevus should be removed is still open to debate, many dermatologists advocate the prophylactic removal of *all* congenital moles greater than ⅗ inch in diameter. Smaller nevi may be photographed and measured, then examined periodically for changes.

NEVUS SEBACEOUS OF JADASSOHN

This tongue twister refers to a sharply bordered, hairless, velvety plaque that is present at birth or develops shortly thereafter. *Nevus sebaceous of Jadassohn* lesions are typically roundish or linear and yellow, yellow-brown, pink, or orange-pink; they range from ¼ inch to over 1 inch in diameter. The scalp and face are favored locations. As a rule, plaques enlarge gradually during early childhood; after puberty, however, they become dramatically thickened, elevated, and nodular.

Nevus sebaceous would be considered just a cosmetic problem did they not, in more than 15 percent of cases, turn malignant sometime during adolescence and adulthood. Although *basal cell skin cancer* is the most common type to develop within a plaque of nevus sebaceous, *squamous cell cancer* and a variety of *sweat gland cancers* may also arise. Rapid enlargement or ulceration of a plaque is a warning sign that malignant changes may be occurring.

Diagnosing nevus sebaceous is usually not difficult. Biopsies are required for confirmation and to determine the presence or absence of malignant changes. Complete surgical excision before puberty is the treatment of choice.

NEUROFIBROMATOSIS

Neurofibromas are soft, smooth, spongy, polyplike growths that appear during childhood or adolescence. They may occur anywhere on the body (usually sparing the palms of the hands and soles of the feet) and may range from ⅛ inch to several inches in diameter. There is usually only one. Although typically flesh colored, neurofibromas are sometimes purplish when small, and pink, blue, or blue-brown when larger. Neurofibromas are benign growths and by themselves are simply cosmetic nuisances.

However, the development of numerous neurofibromas in later childhood and adolescence is a marker for *von Recklinghausen's disease,* a serious, potentially life-threatening condition affecting an estimated 1 in every 3,000 children. Approximately half the instances of this disease are attributed to heredity, the remainder to genetic mutations.

Besides neurofibromas in the skin, other manifestations of von Recklinghausen's include tumors of the nervous system, certain neurologic diseases, and a variety of bone, muscle, ocular, and endocrine abnormalities. In children with neurofibromatosis, malignant changes are estimated to occur in as many as 16 percent of neurofibromas. The presence of at least five medium-sized café au lait spots (see Chapter 5) anywhere on the body, or numerous freckle-sized café au lait spots in the armpits or groin are early clinical clues to the disease.

An isolated neurofibroma in an otherwise healthy child may be either left alone or removed surgically for cosmetic reasons. However, in von Recklinghausen's disease, attention is appropriately focused on the medical problems that must be dealt with; in general, only neurofibromas that are severely disfiguring or impinge on vital organs or structures are surgically excised. Although no cure yet exists for this condition, parents may take some comfort in the fact that many children do not develop the full-blown, multiorgan disease just described. In them, the problems remain confined and manageable. For more information on or referral to medical centers specializing in this condition, you may contact the National Neurofibromatosis Foundation, 141 Fifth Avenue, Suite 7S, New York, NY 10010.

AIDS

At present, there are about 3,000 children suffering from AIDS in the United States alone, and our best estimates suggest that another 20,000 may already be harboring the virus. In children, AIDS is usually contracted in one of three ways: blood transfusions, certain treatments for hemophilia, or birth-related transmission from an infected mother (by far the most common cause). Unfortunately, as heterosexual transmission of the disease becomes increasingly common, we can expect to see even greater numbers of children with AIDS in the not too distant future.

A variety of skin problems have been closely linked to AIDS infection. In general, it is not that AIDS itself causes unique skin diseases; it is more that many ordinary skin conditions tend to persist, recur more frequently, and be more severe, widespread, and harder to treat in AIDS sufferers. These differences reflect the underlying inability of the compromised immune system to handle infection and inflammation properly. At times, a persistent or recurrent skin problem is the first clue to the presence of an underlying immune deficiency disease.

Naturally, abnormal conditions of the skin and mucous membranes are only part of the AIDS problem. The lungs, liver, spleen, lymph nodes, and nervous system may also be involved.

The specific symptoms any child will have depend on the particular organ or organs affected.

Here are some of the more common skin manifestations of AIDS in children. Because they are not unique to AIDS, these conditions are not discussed in detail here. For more on the diagnosis and treatment of a particular problem, consult the appropriate section of this book.

Superficial fungal infections are especially common in AIDS patients. In fact, candida (monilia) infections of the skin and mouth are the most common manifestations of childhood AIDS, with an estimated 50 to 80 percent of children with AIDS suffering from either oral thrush or candida diaper rash (see Chapter 9). Yeast infections of the nails and nail folds are also relatively common. In a setting of immunologic deficiency, yeast diaper rashes tend to recur frequently and may extend well beyond the diaper area, even to the neck. Oral as well as topical therapies are often needed to control these conditions.

In addition to candida, ringworm and athlete's foot fungi (see Chapter 9) are frequent infection producers among children with AIDS. These conditions, too, are more difficult than usual to eradicate and often require prolonged combinations of systemic and topical treatment.

Bacterial and viral infections and mite infestations, which are ordinarily mild in healthy children, tend to be more severe in AIDS patients. Impetigo (usually caused by staph) and cellulitis (usually strep) (see Chapter 9) require aggressive systemic antibiotic treatment in AIDS children to prevent severe complications. Herpes simplex infections of the mouth and lips (run-of-the-mill fever blisters or cold sores) can be particularly virulent in sufferers from AIDS. And the lesions of molluscum contagiosum, another common viral skin disease, may grow unusually large and spread rampantly. Scabies infestations (see Chapter 10), too, can be especially extensive in these children and more difficult to eradicate.

AIDS can also trigger or worsen a variety of common, noninfectious inflammatory conditions and make them more resistant to conventional treatments. Seborrheic dermatitis (see Chapter 7), often limited to the scalp, for example, may in AIDS patients extend to the face and diaper areas. In the same way, outbreaks of widespread, debilitating atopic eczema–like lesions may occur, even in children having no family history of atopy (asthma, hay fever, or eczema). Finally, drug rashes, particularly those caused by sulfa drugs, are also more common in AIDS patients.

At present, the diagnosis and treatment of AIDS requires a team approach including many specialists. For the past couple of years, some improvement in overall health and quality of life has been achieved using the antiviral agent zidovudine (AZT); more recently, another antiviral drug, dideoxyinosine (DDI), has also shown promise. With ongoing research, it is hoped that better preventive measures, specific vaccines, and newer treatments and cures will be developed to defeat this dread epidemic.

STAPHYLOCOCCAL SCALDED SKIN SYNDROME (SSSS)

Staphylococcal scalded skin syndrome, which most often affects children under the age of five, may be thought of as a bullous impetigo (see Chapter 9) run wild. It begins as a tender, red rash, especially prominent around the mouth and nose and in the skin fold areas. Large, flaccid blisters appear all over the body, accompanied by fever and irritability. One or two days later, the blisters break, and extensive areas of skin begin peeling away, resulting in a "scalded skin" appearance. The eruption is caused by a toxin known as *exfoliatin,* which is secreted by several strains of staph organisms harbored in the nose, throat, conjunctiva, or infected wounds. Bacterial cultures help confirm the diagnosis.

In the days before antibiotics, mortality was high among children with this condition. Nowadays, however, with prompt treatment with antistaphylococcal antibiotics, the prognosis is excellent. In many cases (as with burn patients), fluids and salts lost through raw, weeping skin surfaces need to be replaced intravenously. Complete healing generally takes about ten days to two weeks.

VITILIGO

So far, we've covered several serious and even potentially life-threatening skin diseases. Certainly, *vitiligo*, a condition resulting in the patchy loss of normal skin color, would not seem to fit in this chapter. However, the psychological toll this condition may take when it is widespread can be so great that it warrants inclusion here.

Vitiligo affects 1 percent of the American population, and many cases begin in childhood. The tendency for the disorder appears to run in some families. Although its precise cause remains unknown, it is believed to be an autoimmune disease, one of a number of conditions in which the body's immune system goes awry and attacks normal tissue instead of foreign invaders. In this case, healthy melanocytes (the pigment-producing cells of the skin) are the victims.

Vitiligo may affect any area of the body, and pigment loss tends to be symmetrical (meaning, for example, that if the right side of the mouth loses pigment, the left side usually will, too). The face, neck, nostrils, nipples, genitals and other body fold regions, as well as sites of prior skin injury are favored locations. In widespread cases of vitiligo, children can be left with leopard stripe patterns. The psychological impact of this disfigurement cannot be underestimated. Naturally, the darker the child's normal skin, the more obvious the contrast between normal and affected areas.

The course of this condition is variable. Typically, periods of marked disease progression alternate with periods of quiescence.

Although spontaneous improvement occasionally occurs, complete repigmentation is rare.

The diagnosis of vitiligo is usually obvious. In contrast to other depigmenting conditions, such as postinflammatory hypopigmentation (see Chapter 5), when exposed to a Wood's ultraviolet light, areas of vitiligo demonstrate a stark absence of pigment. If the diagnosis remains uncertain, a biopsy may be recommended. The microscopic finding of a complete absence of melanocytes confirms the diagnosis.

There is still no cure for vitiligo. Skin dyes and masking cosmetics (see page 149) can be satisfactory for hiding small areas. For selected cases of more extensive involvement, oral or topical *psoralens* (ultraviolet light–sensitizing medications) coupled with periodic exposure to high-intensity ultraviolet light radiation, a process known as PUVA, can be helpful. In extreme cases, the few remaining islands of normally pigmented skin may be permanently depigmented with monobenzyl ether of hydroquinone (Benoquin). Last but not least, every child with vitiligo must be taught the need for sunscreens and protective clothing to prevent severe sunburns in the depigmented areas. For more information, contact the National Vitiligo Foundation, Inc., Texas American Bank Building, P.O. Box 6337, Tyler, TX 75711.

14

BABIES CAN BE TOUGH ON MOTHER'S SKIN, TOO

This book would be incomplete without at least a brief discussion of the effects that pregnancy and child rearing can have on a mother's skin. Practically from the instant of conception, the developing embryo causes changes in the mother's skin, and after the baby is born, demands on the mother's skin continue. As experienced moms know, everything from nursing and changing diapers to wiping up spills can be tough on their skin. Nevertheless, you will be happy to learn that most skin changes of pregnancy clear up spontaneously after delivery and that most maternal skin problems of the postpregnancy period are preventable or manageable by simple measures.

PHYSIOLOGIC CHANGES
OF PREGNANCY

A number of skin changes occur so frequently during pregnancy that they are considered *physiologic* (normal). In general, they are believed to be related to the massive hormonal surges in the mother's body during this period. Although some effects may be cosmetically disturbing, they are all perfectly harmless.

Hyperpigmentation, or skin darkening, is a regular feature of pregnancy, occurring in as many as 90 percent of women. The changes are generally more pronounced in dark-complexioned women. As a rule, areas of the skin that are normally pigmented will darken most. These include the pink tissue around the nipples *(areolae),* as well as the armpits, inner thighs, vulva, and anus. Preexisting freckles *(ephelides)* and some types of scars and moles *(nevi)* also may darken. The whitish line that extends from the pubic bone to the belly button, the *linea alba,* darkens during pregnancy and is accordingly renamed the *linea nigra.* In general, most pregnancy-related color changes are permanent, although freckles and moles tend to return to their prepregnancy coloration.

Most of these conditions require nothing more than reassurance. However, moles that change in appearance should be looked at by a dermatologist to ensure that nothing more than simple darkening has occurred.

Melasma (often called the mask of pregnancy) is a dramatic form of skin darkening. More frequent in dark-complexioned women, this condition appears to some extent in as many as 50 to 75 percent of all pregnant women and may affect any or all of the following areas: forehead, cheeks, nose, upper lip, and chin. Hormones, sun exposure, and genetics are all felt to play a role. In most cases, the condition fades within a year of delivery. Regular use of sunscreens may prevent the problem. More consistently, sunscreens can be helpful for limiting further discoloration. For treatment, combinations of hydroquinone-containing bleaching preparations (for instance, Melanex) and Retin-A or Lac-Hydrin lotion have been successful in lightening melasma in selected cases. These should be used after delivery, however.

Because tiny blood vessels generally increase in number and size under hormonal stimulation, many kinds of blood vessel changes in the skin occur during pregnancy. *Palmar erythema,* or flushing of the palms, appears in about two-thirds of white women in the first trimester, presumably because of the higher rate and volume of blood flow during this time. In some women, the mottled purple or blotchy reddish coloration characteristic of the condition may extend up the thumbs and wrists. Regardless, the condition is harmless and usually fades within a week of delivery.

Black-and-blue marks *(purpura),* common during the last two trimesters, are believed to be the result of increased capillary fragility and leakage. The appearance may be frightening, but the condition is harmless, and the tendency disappears after delivery. *Cutis marmorata,* or a peculiar episodic bluish mottling of the legs is also common and is believed to be the result of a heightened vascular sensitivity to circulating estrogen. This, too, clears after delivery.

Telangiectasias, or patches of "broken" blood vessels, can appear anywhere, although they commonly occur on the face, neck, shoulders, and back. They are actually dilated (varicose) blood vessels that have lost their ability to contract normally. *Spider nevi,* dilated arterioles with spider leg–like radiations emanating from their centers, affect more than two-thirds of pregnant women. Both telangiectasias and spider nevi generally fade within a few months after delivery. If they persist, your doctor may eliminate them by lightly touching them with a fine electric current, a form of electrolysis.

Cherry hemangiomas, blood blister–like overgrowths of tiny vessels, affect 5 percent of pregnant women during the first trimester.

Varying from purplish to cherry red (hence the name), they may appear anywhere, particularly on the upper chest, abdomen, and back. As pregnancy progresses, they slowly enlarge. Unlike other blood vessel changes, however, most cherry hemangiomas persist after delivery. For cosmetic reasons, they may be removed by simple electrosurgery or a combination of shave excision and electrosurgery (see Chapter 3).

Varicose veins of the legs and *hemorrhoids* (anal varicosities) can become a problem in 40 percent of pregnant women. Increased venous pressure caused by the distended uterus, hormonally me-diated relaxation of blood vessel walls, high blood flow, salt and water retention, and hereditary factors are all felt to contribute to these problems. Fluid retention, or *edema,* is also responsible for swelling of the ankles after prolonged standing and for puffiness in the eyelids and face when arising in the morning.

Although varicose veins of the legs shrink considerably after delivery, they seldom disappear completely. Elevation, support hosiery, and avoidance of prolonged standing, sitting, or excessive weight gain can be helpful. In more troublesome cases, the use of sclerosing agents, which are irritating chemicals injected to close off unwanted vessels, and venous stripping and ligation may be considered after delivery.

Skin tags, soft fleshy flaps of skin, often develop on the face, neck, chest, armpits, groin, and breasts. Although they occasionally disappear following delivery, most enlarge over time. They are easily removable, however, by simple electrosurgery, or by scalpel or scissor excision followed by electrosurgery of the base.

Stretch marks, or *striae gravidarum,* starting from the second trimes-ter on are another common problem, especially in white women. These marks, believed to be caused by tearing or stretching of collagen and elastin fibers, may appear on the breasts and abdo-men and less often on the upper arms, lower back, buttocks, thighs, and in the groin. Beginning as pinkish, wrinkly streaks, they eventually turn whitish lilac or ivory white. Although as a rule they become less noticeable with time, stretch marks are permanent. Creams and lotions marketed to decrease or eliminate them are useless, although the twice daily application of Retin-A after delivery has been found helpful in clearing them up in some cases. Retin-A is not approved for use during pregnancy.

Subtle pregnancy-induced metabolic changes in liver function are felt to be responsible for *idiopathic pruritus* (unexplained itching), also called *pruritus gravidarum* (itching of pregnancy), which affects about 20 percent of women at some point during pregnancy. When metabolic changes in the liver are more pronounced, itching may be accompanied by *physiologic jaundice* (yellowing of the skin and whites of the eyes).

Sometimes the itch concentrates in a small area, usually the abdomen, and is only a minor annoyance; at other times the entire body may be affected, causing severe discomfort. Mild cases of itching can be treated with the regular use of simple hypoallergenic, all-purpose moisturizers (such as Moisturel lotion) to minimize any associated dryness. More severe cases may require topical corticosteroid creams and oral antihistamines to reduce inflammation. Both idiopathic pruritus and physiologic jaundice disappear completely after delivery but may recur with subsequent pregnancies.

Pregnancy also affects the hair. Some women lose hair diffusely or suffer male patternlike hair loss toward the second half of pregnancy. The cause of these conditions is largely unknown. Other women may develop a *postpartum telogen effluvium*, a stress-related hair loss that begins within one to three months following delivery and can continue for several months. In both cases, no therapy other than reassurance is generally needed because complete, spontaneous hair regrowth is the rule.

Some women, particularly those who are dark-complexioned, experience the opposite problem—excessive hair growth *(hirsutism)* during pregnancy. Usually, long, fine, babylike *lanugo* hairs, as well as darker, thicker, *terminal* hairs are produced, commonly appearing on the upper lip, cheeks, and chin. Most of the fine hairs fall out after delivery, but the terminal hairs remain. These may be dealt with in the usual ways: bleaching, tweezing, shaving, and electrolysis. Recurrence of the condition with subsequent pregnancies is common.

Finally, nails can also be affected by pregnancy. Frequently, they may become overly brittle or overly soft. Other changes, such as separation of the nail from the underlying bed and the development of horizontal grooves across the plate, may also develop. Should any of these problems occur, it is best to avoid artificial nails, nail wrapping, and the excessive use of nail polish remover to reduce possible aggravating factors. Fortunately, nail problems of pregnancy usually abate after delivery.

COMMON SKIN PROBLEMS AFTER DELIVERY

The end of pregnancy is often the beginning of a whole new set of skin problems for the parent. Nursing, diaper changes, and other kinds of child care duties all can take their toll.

Nursing can be quite irritating to the nipple and surrounding breast tissue until the breast becomes accustomed to its new task. Soreness, chapping, and painful cracking (*fissuring*) are frequent problems for the new nursing mother. Toward the end of pregnancy, you can help toughen your nipples for the job ahead by gently rubbing them each day. After birth, you may use nipple shields to protect the surrounding area.

Applying moisturizers often helps reduce irritation. However, be sure to wipe the nipple areas thoroughly clean of any product applied before nursing. Immediately after nursing, cleanse the breasts gently and reapply the moisturizer.

Soreness and redness over an area of the breast, especially if accompanied by fever, may signal infection or a breast abscess.

Prompt treatment of these conditions is required to prevent complications. Warm compresses and oral antibiotics are usually indicated, but nursing seldom needs to be discontinued, even temporarily. The infection generally responds rapidly to therapy. Check with your child's pediatrician about this.

Hand dermatitis, sometimes referred to as *housewife's eczema,* is another common accompaniment to new parenthood. Diaper changes, which expose your skin to the highly irritating effects of urine and stool, and frequent hand washings can take their toll. Other wet work (such as cleaning dishes and spills) compounds the problem. Hands can become dry, red, rough, and painfully cracked. Without proper care, eczema and infection may develop. Parents with a personal or family history of eczema are particularly prone to these conditions.

To prevent these problems, try wearing white cotton gloves for dry work (dusting) and white cotton gloves under vinyl overgloves for wet work (dishes, diapers). These can be picked up at a local surgical supply store or ordered from Allerderm Laboratories (Mill Valley, CA 94941). If you find gloves too annoying or difficult to use for diaper changes (disposable diaper tapes usually catch on the gloves), you might try using tongs to lift diapers and to reduce direct contact with moisture, urine, and stool.

Some harried parents might laugh at the impracticality of using tongs and putting on and taking off gloves dozens of times a day. Nevertheless, you should attempt to do everything practical to preserve your hands. Other suggestions include switching to gentle soapless soaps or sensitive skin cleansers (for example, Lowila Cake or Moisturel sensitive skin cleanser) and moisturizing your hands immediately after each cleansing. For added protection, especially when changing diapers, you might find commercial barrier creams (for instance, Wonder Glove or Dermaffin) more practical, against not only moisture but a variety of other irritating substances. Such products have been formulated to withstand repeated hand washings. A potent moisturizer, such as Lac-

Hydrin lotion (available by prescription only), between washings might also prove useful, especially for individuals with sensitive or eczema-prone skin.

Fingernails, too, may suffer the effects of new parenthood. Chronic exposure to moisture and irritants may lead to brittleness and splitting. And damage to cuticles can leave the folds surrounding the nails ragged and susceptible to certain infections, particularly yeast infection. This condition is especially likely if your baby is suffering from a yeast diaper rash.

To keep them protected, nails may be coated with a clear polish. Avoid excessive manicuring, artificial nails, or overtrimming the cuticles. To strengthen nails and replenish their natural moisture content, try soaking them in plain, tepid water for a few minutes each night, then applying a potent urea- or lactic acid–containing moisturizer (for example, Lac-Hydrin 5) to the nails and surrounding skin immediately after patting dry.

Finally, several other skin problems are more indirectly related to the new baby in the home. Lack of sleep and the increasing demands on your time make it increasingly hard for you to take care of yourself properly. As a result, dark circles and puffiness may begin showing under your eyes, and your complexion may become sallow. In addition, the new stresses in your life may trigger old problems, such as acne, psoriasis, or eczema. It is therefore imperative for you to set aside time for yourself for proper rest and relaxation. Eating and exercising regularly, napping while your baby naps, and taking time to care for your own skin problems are essential for your skin's health and appearance. You *can* look as radiant as you did before the baby came along. Keep in mind that you must take care of yourself in order to be at your best for your baby. And that, too, is an important part of infant and child care.

INDEX

SPF (sun protection factor), 17
Spider bites, 125–26
Spider nevi, 167
Spitz nevi, 54–55
Sprays, 35
Staphylococcal scalded skin
  syndrome, 161–62
Staphylococcus aureus, 144
Stevens-Johnson syndrome, 98
Stomatitis, aphthous, 109
Stork bite, 40
Stratum corneum, 24
Stratum spinosum, 24
Strawberry hemangiomas, 150–51
Strawberry tongue, 106
Stress-induced hair loss, 137–38
Stretch marks, 168–69
Striae gravidarum, 168–69
Subcutis, 25
Subungual hematoma, 142–43
Sucking blisters, 38
Sudamina, 44
Summertime pityriasis, 85
Sunglasses, 18, 19
Sun protection, 13–20
Sunscreens, 16–18
Superfatted soaps, 5
Superficial folliculitis, 103
Supernumerary appendages, 48
Surfactants, 4
  amphoteric, 7
Sweat glands, 25
  cancer of, 157
Systemic medications, 36

Tactile contact, *ix*
Talcum powders, 11
Target lesion, 98
Telangiectasias, 167
Telangiectatic nevi, 40
Telogen effluvium, 137–38
  postpartum, 169
Telogen phase, 136

Terminal hairs, 169
Thrush, 116
Ticks, 123–25
Tics, hair-pulling, 140–41
Tidemark dermatitis, 65
Tineas, 117–19
Toilet soaps, 4
Topical anesthetics, 29–30
Topical medications, 34, 35
Toxic erythema, 41–42
Traction alopecia, 140
Transient neonatal pustular
  melanosis, 42–43
Trichorrhexis nodosa, 141
Trichotillomania, 140–41
Tumor, 28
Tzanck smears, 108

Ulcers, 27
Ultras, 10, 11
Ultraviolet radiation, 14, 15, 19
Urticaria, 94–96
  papular, 133–34

Varicella, 112–13
Varicose veins, 168
Vascular birthmarks, 147
Vascular nevi, 147
Vernix caseosa, 37
Verrucae, 109–11
Vesicles, 28
Viral infections, 106–12, 160
Vitiligo, 162–63
von Recklinghausen's disease, 59,
  158–59

Warts, 109–11
  water, 112
Washable lotions, 5
Wasps, 129
Water warts, 112
Wheals, 29, 94–96
White blood cells, 26